"I have known Michael for over two decades, and throughout that time I have admired his vision, expertise, and dedication to advancing our profession. When he shared his idea for a book on best practices in clinical data management, I immediately saw the value it could bring to the industry and was honored to be invited to contribute as a reviewer. As a long-standing leader in the Society for Clinical Data Management (SCDM), Michael has a unique perspective on the evolving needs of our field. This book will serve as a much-needed, practical guide for ensuring high-quality, on-time clinical data deliverables – an essential part of bringing new treatments to patients around the world. I wish him great success in bringing this important work to publication".

Jonathan Andrus, *Co-CEO, CRIO & Treasurer, SCDM*

"I had the pleasure of reporting to Michael when we both worked at PRA/ ICON. We built a strong relationship during that tenure and continue to stay in touch to exchange new perspectives in our industry. I was very excited when Michael mentioned to me earlier about his idea to put together a book on best practices in clinical data management. The industry is lacking a concise guide at this stage, and this reference book will fill a much-needed gap in clinical data management. I felt honored when Michael invited me to write a chapter for the book.

As one of the leaders in the Society for Clinical Data Management (SCDM), the clinical data management industry's recognized forum for nurturing best practices, Michael has a unique lens into the needs of the industry. I am confident that the book he is striving to get published will assist personnel in the industry in practicing end-to-end data management steps that will ensure on-time, high-quality deliverables. Clinical Data Management deliverables will be a key factor in bringing much-needed cures to patients worldwide".

Zia Haque, *Head of Data Management at Otsuka-US Pharmaceuticals*

"As Chief Data strategist and solutions officer I see too many companies not fully understanding the importance and value in their data. This starts with having a better understanding of best practices in data management, and where clinical data science is taking us as an industry. With publications like this book, written by experts such as Michael, which brings the data delivery and quality aspects to life through easy reading (including practical examples), the industry is one step closer to getting true value out of their data".

Tanya du Plessis, *Bioforum*

Mastering Clinical Data Management

Clinical Research is a fascinating industry, because 99.9% of human beings interact with it throughout their lives. However, very few understand the effort to bring a new medical product to patients in need, and an even smaller number have thought about, or remotely understand, the pivotal role Clinical Data Management (CDM) professionals play in this endeavor. Ranging from sharing hands-on experiences to providing concrete examples of how to propel one's CDM career, *Mastering Clinical Data Management: The Background, Experience, and Soft Skills Needed to Succeed in CDM* is a glimpse of the author's three-decade-long experience in the field.

Decentralized Clinical Trials (DCTs), Risk-Based Quality Management (RBQM), examining the trustworthiness of the data used in clinical research, or illustrating the use of Artificial Intelligence (AI) in CDM are just a few examples of topics this book not only covers, but also explains for all competency levels through real-life examples. Despite Clinical Research in general, and the profession of CDM in particular, being a heavily regulated and tech-driven environment, this book uses every opportunity to emphasize the importance of the human in the loop. Therefore, in addition to gaining more insights into the fascinating world of CDM, this book provides the perfect "How to" of advancing one's career and learning the art of CDM.

The goal is to provide valuable insights for all levels of CDM professionals and those individuals that might consider a career in CDM.

Key Features

- Provides insight into clinical data and its importance as never seen before
- Draws on 35 years of hands-on CDM experience
- Provides guidance and many examples of crucial soft skills needed to succeed in CDM
- Provides arguments for all CDMs to excel in their current work environment
- Reflects on the current regulatory framework and how it can benefit CDM

Michael Goedde is Certified Clinical Data Manager with 35 years of experience in the pharmaceutical and biotechnology industry. His expertise ranges from hands-on clinical data management (CDM) activities to executive roles with responsibility for large international teams and strategic positioning for the companies he engages with. Michael has dedicated his professional career to the advancement of CDM as a recognized and respected profession in our industry, as well as providing mentoring for the next generation of CDM enthusiasts.

Mastering Clinical Data Management

The Background, Experience, and Soft Skills Needed to Succeed in CDM

Michael Goedde

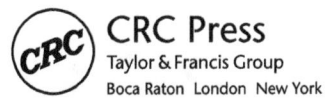

CRC Press
Taylor & Francis Group
Boca Raton   London   New York

CRC Press is an imprint of the
Taylor & Francis Group, an **informa** business

A CHAPMAN & HALL BOOK

Designed cover image: David Fornos – guindillasmedia

First edition published 2026
by CRC Press
2385 NW Executive Center Drive, Suite 320, Boca Raton FL 33431

and by CRC Press
4 Park Square, Milton Park, Abingdon, Oxon, OX14 4RN

CRC Press is an imprint of Taylor & Francis Group, LLC

© 2026 Michael Goedde

ISBN: 978-1-041-09072-4 (hbk)
ISBN: 978-1-041-08690-1 (pbk)
ISBN: 978-1-003-64831-4 (ebk)

DOI: 10.1201/9781003648314

Typeset in Palatino
by Apex CoVantage, LLC

Contents

Introduction and Acknowledgments

Clinical Research is a fascinating industry, because 99.9% of human beings interact with it from day 1 of their lives and continue to do so for all the years to come thereafter. From pain relievers, over vaccines, to life-saving medicines, most of us have either direct or indirect experiences of how these products can improve people's lives – or not.

However, only a very small number of people understand the effort to bring a new medical product to patients in need, and an even smaller number have thought about, or remotely understand, the pivotal role Clinical Data Management (CDM) professionals play in this endeavor.

Mastering Clinical Data Management is a small glimpse of my 3+ decades-long experience in the field, ranging from sharing hands-on experiences to providing concrete examples of how to propel one's CDM career. Most importantly though, my goal is to provide valuable insights for all levels of CDM professionals and those individuals that might consider a career in CDM.

The main reason for me to write this book is to show that despite the CDM profession being part of a heavily regulated industry and bound to follow rigorous scientific standards, one key element of success, which keeps on being forgotten in the currently available literature, is to show the importance of the human element in the loop. Spoiler alert – CDM is not an exact science. It is a form of art!

Therefore, entire chapters and many examples focus on cultural aspects within companies, required soft skills of CDM professionals, and the more subjective and experience-based skill sets required to ensure state-of-the-art CDM execution and value creation.

It is my hope, with this book, to inspire current professionals to become more outspoken advocates for CDM and the importance of reliable clinical data overall, as well as to encourage the next generation of to-be Clinical Data Managers to get excited about the abundant carrier opportunities and rewarding accomplishments this profession has to offer.

I am very thankful that a long chain of coincidences, plenty of luck, and mentors who took the time to share their experiences with me all along resulted in allowing me to experience the joys of making a career in CDM.

Another fact of our industry, despite being global and large, is the amazing network of like-minded colleagues and friends that can be built over time. It is this network that I tapped into to help me get this book going and finished.

It is my absolute privilege to thank and acknowledge first and foremost the individuals who helped review some of the chapters. Hugh Donovan, my life-long professional and personal mentor, without whom I undoubtedly would never have found my voice in the CDM community.

Jonathan Andrews, who some refer to as "Mr. CDM" and who has been an inspiration to me on how he relentlessly and eloquently has been positively influencing the standing of CDM in the last 20 years through his record tenure on the Board of Trustees for the Society for Clinical Data Management (SCDM) and countless presentations at industry venues.

And Tanya du Plessis, a current Board of Trustees member for SCDM and expert in many specialized areas of CDM, such as the regulatory framework, RBQM, and others. She pairs her knowhow with such contagious energy and enthusiasm, which makes her simply irresistible.

Hugh, Jonathan, and Tanya, thank you so much for the time dedicated for your respective reviews and input!

In addition to the aforementioned reviewers and with the intent to not solely rely on my points of view, I want to recognize the main contributors of some of the chapters for this book. These individuals can also look back on decades of experience in the industry on top of unique subject matter expertise in specific areas.

Joanna Florek-Marwitz and Osnat Mamet for their contributions for the "Demystifying Risk-Based Quality Management (RBQM) and Why CDM Should Lead It" chapter,

Zia Haque for the "Technology Overload: How to Avoid Common Pitfalls" chapter,

Stephen Cameron for the "Clinical Data Management versus Clinical Data Science" chapter,

and Emily Mitchell for spearheading the content of the "Demystifying DCTs (Decentralized Clinical Trials)" chapter.

Without your contributions, authorship, and continuous encouragement, dear Joanna, Osnat, Zia, Stephen, and Emily, fundamental elements of this book would not have been possible. Thank you!

Not as a contributor, but surely as facilitator and motivator, I have and want to thank Amir Malka, founder and CEO of my current employer, for his support and patience with me to allow me the time to work on this book, despite our pretty full work agenda. Thank you, Amir!

This book includes a good number of graphical representations and pictures. Another big Thank You to Gefen Shen, who despite my last-minute request was able to turn many of my draft outlines into much more appealing visuals. Thank you, Gefen!

As another last-minute rescuer, I also want to thank David Fornos from the guindillasmedia graphic design team (guindillasmedia.com) who was able to adjust the images to the required format and created the really cool and eye-catching cover image. Thank you, David!

I also want to extend my deepest gratitude and respect for Taylor & Francis, in the person of David Grubbs, the Senior Editor for this project and the invaluable guidance and expertise provided to get this project off the ground and finished.

Most importantly, I want to thank my wife, Sònia, for her support and encouragement all along. I do know that I am deeply indebted to her, because of all the off-work hours I was not able to dedicate to her and the family but spent on researching and advancing this dear-to-my-heart book project. Thank you, and I promise to make it up to you, Sònia.

Lastly, I also want to take the opportunity to dedicate this book, my first one, to my parents Montserrat Fornos Rossell and Ortwin Goedde, as their love and dedication were the original building blocks for the development of my values, priorities, and courage to speak up when needed.

Thank you, Mama, your strength and wisdom are still and will always be my inspiration; and Papa, may you rest in peace, thank you for showing me the importance of respect, fairness, and honesty.

About the Contributors

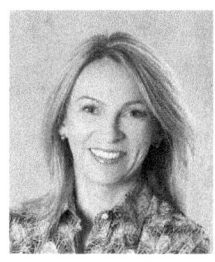

Joanna Florek-Marwitz

Joanna has over 20 years of managerial and technical experience in the clinical research industry delivering business and data transformation solutions. She has extensive experience in clinical and non-interventional trials operations across all therapeutic areas and is an expert in clinical data management, integrated risk-based quality management, innovation, and change management methodologies driving operational efficiencies.

Her technical experience and background in analytics and process improvement have brought critical value to technology implementations focused on patient safety and reliable data in accordance with the current regulatory framework for risk-based approaches.

With her expertise and enthusiasm, Joanna leads new ways of working with clinical data, knowing that the growing scale of accumulated data requires us to establish an entirely new relationship with it.

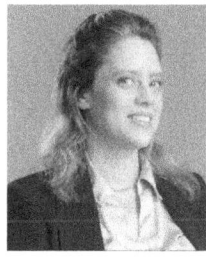

Osnat Mamet

Osnat Mamet is VP of Quality Assurance & IT, with more than 12 years of experience in the pharmaceutical industry. She has extensive expertise in quality management systems, GCP, cGMP, GDP, and regulatory compliance, and has successfully led numerous IT and compliance initiatives across clinical supply operations and data-driven environments.

Previously, Osnat held senior quality management roles in clinical supply services and worked within global compliance functions, gaining broad exposure to international regulatory expectations and cross-functional collaboration. She holds a B.Sc. in Life Sciences and an MBA and is passionate about fostering a strong culture of quality, innovation, and operational excellence across organizations.

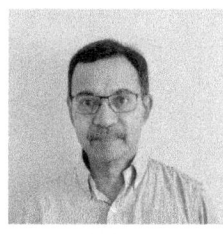

Zia Haque

Zia Haque is a motivational leader in clinical data management with an operations and people management tenure spanning across 28 years. Following roles of increased responsibility with leading Clinical Research Organizations, he is presently serving as Head of Data Management for a pharmaceutical sponsor organization.

His expertise includes identifying, creating, and implementing department-level data management strategies, fostering collaborative team environments, and driving innovation in clinical data management processes and technology. Zia is enthusiastic about mentoring and developing talent while ensuring quality and compliance in all aspects of clinical data management.

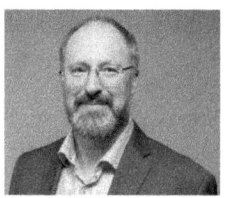

Stephen Cameron

Stephen has close to 30 years of biotechnology, microbiology, and clinical trial data management experience. His areas of focus include recombinant, subunit, attenuated, and whole cell bacterin and viral vaccines, cellular therapy, oncology, gout, and biosimilar studies as well as monoclonal therapies. He has significant exposure to global team leadership, project management, and data operations functional management support for local and global team members, including clinical data coordinators, clinical data scientists, and people leaders. He is also an active member of the Society for Clinical Data Management (SCDM) including tenures as conference co-chair, Board of Trustees, and the Executive Board as well as numerous global presentations and educational engagements on the practice of innovative, cutting-edge, and regulatory compliant clinical data management.

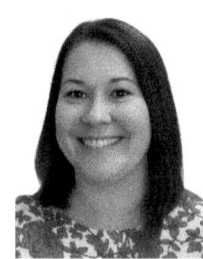

Emily Mitchell

Emily Mitchell is a seasoned Decentralized Clinical Trial (DCT) expert who combines strategic thinking with hands-on expertise to drive innovation and results. With several years of experience working at the intersection of digital strategy, content creation, and technology implementation, Emily has consistently delivered measurable impact, be it optimizing workflow through automation, enhancing brand presence online, or leading cross-functional teams in high-growth environments.

Emily holds a background in CRO and technology operational management and has worked in roles spanning all phases of research and multiple indications. She is passionate about leveraging DCT to enable meaningful connections, minimizing patients' burden, and empowering organizations to thrive in an increasingly digital world.

1

The Role of CDM in Clinical Research and Why It Matters

Introducing the Role of CDM in Clinical Research

In this first chapter we dive into the often misunderstood and underestimated world of Clinical Data and the professionals tasked to take care of it.

We start by showing the unique value Clinical Data has in Clinical Research and why putting it at the center of attention is needed to ensure successful execution of Clinical Trials. After setting the baseline for Clinical Data we will have a detailed look at the most prominent roles and their responsibilities within Clinical Data Management (CDM), followed by examining key deliverables of CDM and sharing best-practice approaches for successful cross-functional implementation.

In addition to providing the baseline understanding and take-off point for all subsequent chapters, the examples, provocative comparisons, and unique perspective of the CDM components presented will already allow you to derive some valuable conclusions for your CDM environment. The aim is to start leaving behind the often-seen inferiority complex within CDM and allow us to imagine Clinical Research with CDM on center stage.

In this chapter, we will cover the following topics:

- "Clinical Data" – The most valuable asset in Clinical Research
- Roles in CDM – Embracing Accountability
- CDM Deliverables
- CDM Driving Cross-Functional Work and Excellence

"Clinical Data" – The Most Valuable Asset in Clinical Research

Daily news headlines originating from biotech and pharmaceutical companies proudly announcing positive results, on the one hand, from a Clinical

Trial often read like this: "Biotech/Pharma company X today announced positive topline results for its study of experimental new drug Y, showing a statistically significant efficacy improvement over the comparator, with a p-value of <0.0001 while achieving a comparable (or improved) safety profile . . .".

On the other hand, when the results are not favorable, the headline will include a phrase indicating that the experimental drug either failed to show a statistically significant improvement in efficacy or had an unfavorable safety profile (i.e., adverse events [AEs] outweighing the possible benefit of the new drug), or both.

These headlines represent the culmination and final result of a clinical trial after years of work done by clinical research teams and millions of US dollars spent. The results can represent the green light for a New Drug Application (NDA)/Biologics License Application (BLA) to the FDA, the advancement of the clinical program to the next stage with more clinical trials, or, for the negative case, the end of the development for this compound overall, or in part for a given dose, method of administration, or indication.

The impact of clinical trial results for the Biotech and Pharma companies working on them is massive. It often triggers, for publicly traded companies, significant stock price moves in either direction. They can also be the catalyst for more funding money, expansions in all areas, and making companies more attractive for M&A (Merger and Acquisition) activities. Beyond the valid business-related interests for successful execution of clinical trials, the main goal remains to increase the understanding of diseases, while continuing the journey to investigate new approaches to increase quality of life for patients through the approval of new medicines.

Let us now have a look behind the scenes and discover one area of clinical research that is, for the most part, undervalued and misunderstood – CDM.

It should be obvious that in order to be able to interpret and report on results that will directly impact patients' lives, and the success, or the lack thereof, for life science companies, the underlying clinical data to support any scientific claim has to conform with the highest standards of integrity possible.

So how is it possible that the profession of CDM, even after decades of being a key enabling factor in the effort of bringing new medical products to market, does not have, for the most part, the same standing, acknowledgement, and recognition compared to the colleagues in Clinical Operations, Biostatistics, Medical Review, or any other typical role represented in a Clinical Study Team? How can it be that there are still companies, mostly on the smaller Biotech side, which do not even have an actual CDM department as part of their organization, and what should be default CDM tasks are handled by IT, Programmers, or Clinical representatives that have a knack for data?

It is important to understand the multitude of reasons for this widespread misconception of CDM, in order to recognize it, address it, and fix it within your respective company.

In my opinion, it starts with the word "Clinical" in the description of the Profession of "Clinical Data Management", or "Clinical Data Science" as the next evolutionary step for CDM, or prominent role names within the CDM department such as "Lead Clinical Data Manager" or "Clinical Data Coordinator". For many companies, both for Biotech/Pharma and for Service Providers, the word "Clinical" is omitted from the department name and/or from the different CDM role names. This results in organizational charts showing "Data Management" or "Data Operations" next to the departments of "Clinical Operations", "Pharmacovigilance", or "Medical Directors", as well as the respective roles being listed as "Lead Data Manger", "Data Coordinator", compared to role names from the other functions being described as "Clinical Study Coordinator", "Clinical Research Associate", "Clinical Program Manager", and so on. How misleading and absurd the omission of the word "Clinical" for CDM is, can be seen, if we look at how other functions and roles would sound, if they were treated the same way. "Clinical Operations" would just be "Operations"! Operations of what? "Clinical Research Associates" would just be "Research Associates"! Researching what?

The omission of the word "Clinical" for CDM has unfortunately even more severe implications for the people working within CDM roles resulting in career disadvantages and below market compensation. During the periodic merit adjustment cycles at companies, where I was leading CDM Teams, a typical argument with my colleagues in Human Resources would circle around agreeing on fair salary range benchmarks for CDM professionals. A common error was to use industry benchmarks for CDM role names without the word "Clinical" in it, resulting in finding salary ranges for all sorts of "Data Management" professionals from other industries, such as banking, IT/Tech companies, or retail sales, which for the most part have significant lower salary ranges than their counterparts in the "Clinical" Research space.

When narrowing the focus of the argument around the importance of the consistent use of the word "Clinical" within CDM departments, it comes down to the simple fact that "Clinical Data Management" is very different from just "Data Management" in its scope and required skill set. I am certain there is no ill intent from representatives of other functions omitting the "Clinical" part. However, stripping away the word "Clinical" automatically narrows the expected deliverables from the "Data Management" Department to the more technical items, such as database builds, edit check programming, and running listing outputs for Clinical/Medical Review. This completely negates the full value and scope that "Clinical Data Management" can and should bring to the table as an, at least, equal member of a clinical study or project team.

However, before falling too much into what could be interpreted as the CDM victim role, let me shed some light on how CDM professionals themselves can be their worst enemies on the journey toward earning and deserving equal respect and recognition. One expression that is being used constantly within Clinical Research to describe the sentiment around CDM is that of being a "Black Box". On the one hand, from the outside the other functional representatives might not fully grasp the different roles and responsibilities the CDM function entails. On the other hand, there is often not enough outgoing educational information and active participation in cross-functional meetings and attempts to open the "CDM Black Box" coming from within CDM either. A common approach in successful CDM departments is the proactive outreach of the department heads, or other vocal and confident representatives from CDM, to their respective cross-functional colleagues. Examples of how to engage with other functions are as follows: inviting other departmental representatives to CDM town hall meetings, volunteering to present CDM topics at the town hall or departmental meetings from other functions, or sharing relevant information that was obtained through industry conference attendance or actual in-house case studies, on the CDM intranet page of the respective company.

You might wonder why it is of such paramount importance for CDM to be understood by others, and for CDM professionals to proactively embrace their lead roles within a Clinical Study/Project Team? Well, the importance of the correct distribution of responsibilities and tasks can be easily derived by constantly having the actual and ultimate goal of running a Clinical Study within a Clinical Program in mind. This goal being the delivery of proof for the hypotheses to show clinically relevant benefits from new investigational medical products for the general populations, compared to the current standard of care. And what is the fundamental ingredient for any sort of hypothesis testing? You got it – Trustworthy Clinical Data! Or in other words, clinical data that reflects reality, is unadulterated, is authentic, can be fully traced back to its source, is complete, or has any other characteristic you want to tag on, which can describe the desire and mandate to only approve those new medical products that possess an actual benefit, and block the ones, which do not, or could even cause harm.

Following this train of thought, it puts many of the efforts and resources that Biotech and Pharma companies invest into the execution of clinical trials into perspective. As an example, items that are usually a given in any clinical study and consume large part of any clinical budget, such as clinical site identification, recruiting patients into clinical trials, or sending Clinical Research Associates (CRAs) to sites to perform Source Data Review (SDR) and Source Data Verification (SDV), are ultimately only being done to collect clinical data. Looking at clinical trials not through the lenses of different functions executing such trials, but focusing on the true purpose, or dare I say reason for their existence, which is the gathering of evidence in the form of clinical data, suddenly does shift the spotlight more toward the custodians and accountable individuals of this data, which are the CDM professionals. In no form should this way of describing the cross-functional effort of planning, conducting, and finishing a clinical study diminish the value that all functions bring to the table. It would, in fact, be almost impossible to successfully execute a clinical study without the respective subject matter input of all functions.

Let us look at a theoretical example to emphasize again the center stage role clinical data should have. If reliable clinical data were available to a Biotech or Pharma company without having to run a clinical trial and be able to prove or disprove the hypotheses of their planned clinical studies, they could go directly to the finish line of a given project without the need for Sites, Patients, Clinical Study Teams, and all related functions, as they would be rendered obsolete. Interestingly enough, this example is not as far-fetched or hypothetical as it might seem. The use of so-called "Synthetic Arms" has been on the rise in recent years, as some Biotech and Pharma companies have identified opportunities to use either broadly accepted historic data from the literature or existing outcomes from the real-world use of certain medications. This approach has shown that time and money can be saved, by not having to use a comparator arm at all or possibly reduce the number of patients in the comparator arm(s). This approach allows either for more patients actually receiving the experimental product, or for fewer patients to be enrolled into the study overall. The argument being made here is that for the clinical data originating from a synthetic arm, other than ensuring the robustness of the source, statistical considerations around comparability of data from these distinct sources, and some regulatory considerations, not much involvement is required by any other function.

Some might find it provocative to claim that clinical data is the most valuable asset in clinical research and wonder about all the other important factors required to bring a new medical product to market. As an example, there are patients who volunteer for clinical studies. There is, rightly so, a lot of talk and emphasis on patient centricity and the mandatory safeguards that must be in place to ensure patients' safety and wellbeing throughout the full conduct of a study. These patients are the targeted "customers" for the new experimental medical product. Without patients' volunteering there could not be clinical studies, and therefore it is encouraging to see an increased effort to democratize clinical studies, to ensure greater diversification of patient populations, and to make it easier for patients to be aware and participate in studies that can possibly provide lifesaving alternatives to the standard of care options provided.

Another obvious prerequisite is the existence of the Investigational Product (IP) itself. It takes years of laboratory work, enabled by huge pre-clinical R&D investments, to identify promising new medical solutions that can be brought into the clinical setting and are deemed safe for use in humans.

However, when we try to find the common denominator around contributing factors toward a successful clinical program, such as patients, IP, decade-long assignment of 100s of cross-functional team members, and overall investments in the billions of US dollars, we see that the actual life-blood, the common language spoken, and the true currency of the clinical research industry is Clinical Data!

Yes, we deeply care about the patients in our clinical studies, want them to do well, and ultimately benefit from more and better healthcare options.

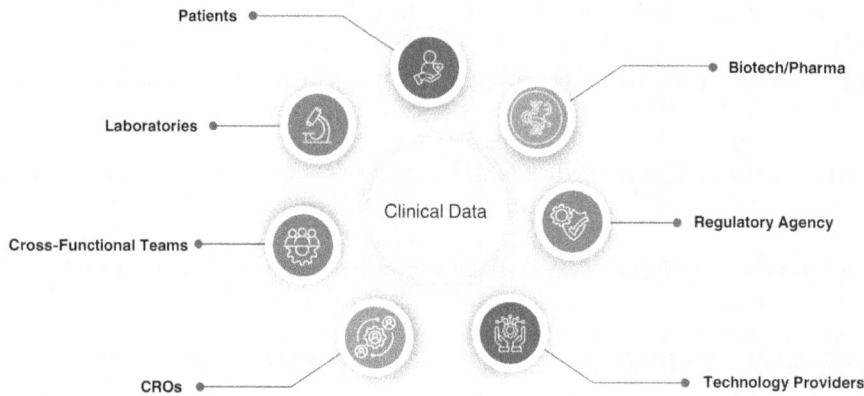

FIGURE 1.1
Clinical Data – Center of focus in our industry.

And how do we do this? We collect every data point pertaining to these patients, as defined in the clinical protocol, to identify any risk as soon as possible and to support the underlying hypothesis of a given study.

When looking at the aforementioned cross-functional teams, which often represent different companies such as the technology sector, CROs, laboratories, the sponsor company itself, or our colleagues at Regulatory Agencies, we realize that the way these individuals actually communicate is through the exchange, presentation, and interpretation of clinical data.

The inherent complexity of the ins and outs of the decade-long process behind medical advances driven by the clinical research industry can be overwhelming even for industry veterans. There is still the unmet need to define the North Star of our combined efforts industrywide. It is time to step up to the plate for CDM professionals and declare Clinical Data to be the North Star on our never-ending journey toward bettering human lives.

Roles in CDM – Embracing Accountability

Introduction to Roles in CDM

Now that we have established the foundation for the crucial importance of robust Clinical Data in Clinical Research, let us have a closer look into the people and roles that are accountable for it. We will look at:

- Lead (Clinical) Data Manager (LDM)/Clinical Data Science Lead (CDSL)
- Database Designer (DD)/Clinical System Lead (CSL)

- Testers
- Clinical Data Coordinator (CDC)
- Other (e.g., Clinical Coder [CC], CDM/SDTM Programmer)

These role descriptions will illustrate the breadth of reach CDM should have in every clinical research company.

I am using the word "should", as in my experience, due to prevailing misconceptions and organizational structures in the Clinical Research industry, CDM continues to be too often an afterthought in the conduct of clinical studies. The voices of CDM professionals in Clinical Study Team Meetings do not seem to have the gravitas they need to have. We will investigate reasons for this dilemma from multiple angles and explore ways to find a way out of it throughout this book.

Before tackling the more challenging discussion on how to embrace accountability as a CDM professional and take a step toward leading study and project teams through the clinical data jungle, we will look at the actual roles within CDM.

I cannot claim that the CDM role names I am suggesting are being used and interpreted the same way universally, but I will be sharing what I have observed over the last three decades across CROs, Technology, Biotech, and Pharma companies while sharing the most commonly used wordings and descriptions. One additional complexity is the rapid pace of change seen in CDM and the industry in general. In addition to the constantly evolving environment, even farther-reaching factors, such as the advances in artificial intelligence (AI) and machine learning (ML) globally, are heavily shaking and questioning the foundations of long-established beliefs and practices.

Lastly, we must also consider the ongoing evolutionary transformation from CDM to Clinical Data Science (CDS), which was jumpstarted by the COVID pandemic, the acceptance of decentralized clinical trial approaches, and the supporting changes in the regulatory guidance framework.

The LDM

Let us start with the most visible role in CDM – the *LDM*. Other names I have seen for this role are Study Data Manager (SDM), or for program-level oversight it can be Project Data Manager (PDM). More recent variations for this role can also include the "Data Science" component, which then results in role names such as *Clinical Data Science Lead (CDSL)*. The latter variation provides a hint that the CDM department for this company has at least embarked on the journey toward expanding CDM into the Data Science field or is already at the stage of fully having performed the transformation to a data-driven approach for the company led by CDM professionals.

Either way, for the moment we will use LDM as the most commonly used role name by which we identify the person accountable for all CDM activities for a given clinical study. The area of responsibility can vary slightly, depending on the company the LDM works for. At a sponsor company (i.e., Biotech or Pharma), the LDM role typically includes oversight tasks, in case CDM deliverables have been outsourced to a CRO.

On the CRO side, however, LDMs often have to cover a few more administrative tasks such as overseeing budgetary items, performing resource planning, or presenting at bid-defense meetings and providing input for client proposals. The interpretation of the role can also differ regarding the level of detail LDMs operate. At some companies it can be a pure Project Management assignment, where LDMs' main task is to develop and oversee the Project Plan and Timelines for all CDM-related activities and ensure that quality- and performance-related metrics are established and acted on, thus basically acting as a CDM Project Manager. In this scenario LDMs are delegating tasks to more hands-on CDM roles and do not get too close to the Clinical Data they are ultimately accountable for.

On the other side of the spectrum, you have LDMs that actively look at Clinical Data, review specifications, provide input into data review strategies, and have a deeper understanding and connection with the Clinical Data. Using a more hands-on approach for LDMs also results in a smaller number of clinical studies LDMs work on simultaneously, because of the more in-depth knowledge these professionals must represent in cross-functional meetings intra- and intercompany wide.

Regardless of one's interpretation of the LDM role and where individuals land on the spectrum of "detailed involvement" to "high-level", the most important commonality for the LDM is the mandate to take ownership and full accountability for all CDM deliverables. Even though we will explore in more detail the most relevant and impactful deliverables for CDM in the next part, we should at least set the stage here, when talking about LDM responsibilities.

It starts with the review and input for the Clinical Protocol, or its synopsis, albeit it being a deliverable authored and owned by Clinical Operations and the Medical Director. The LDM should evaluate the clinical data described in the protocol and check for redundancies or gaps, as well as ensuring that the description is specific enough to allow for unambiguous data collection. The Protocol also serves as the key reference for LDMs to estimate over CDM efforts in terms of resource needs and complexity, as the protocol will provide information related to the size, in terms of patients and clinical sites, and length of the study, in terms of the number of visits or cycles. The biggest impact on complexity, however, is not driven by the size or length of the study but is directly related to the number of distinct data sources. How many different laboratories, electronic patient-reported outcomes (ePRO), or decentralized data collection methods need to be accounted for by the LDM, in addition to the default electronic data capture (EDC) and interactive response technology (IRT) source? Knowing full well that each of these sources will require their own data transfer specification (DTS) and testing.

Furthermore, the LDM should be able to derive the number of unique and repeat data domains, as well as the extent that Data Standards can be used.

After ensuring that CDM input has been considered in the Clinical Protocol development process, the focus shifts to the area of preparing for Clinical Data Collection, Clinical Data Review, and the initiation of the central document in CDM, the (Clinical) Data Management Plan (DMP).

Working hand in hand with the Clinical Database Designer, which we will introduce next, the LDM ensures that all required data collection instruments (DCIs), which include more than just the EDC system, are ready for deployment shortly before one of the most prominent milestones in clinical research – First Patient In (FPI). Whether FPI truly deserves the hype and spotlight it usually gets by different stakeholders is questionable. It is important to bear in mind that quite often the main motivation for forcing acceleration of FPI timelines is driven primarily by publicity considerations of companies eager to get a press release announcing to the world the actual start of the study. Of course, there is nothing wrong per se with wanting to accelerate any step on the journey to bring possibly new life improving medicines to market. Accelerated FPI is often only achieved by focusing on activating one clinical site which has one patient in the screening queue. It might then take weeks, or even months, to get a second patient enrolled in this study with no time gained toward the much more relevant milestone of Last Patient Out (LPO), which actually triggers the final clinical data collection and reviews efforts toward database lock and data analysis.

This little side tangent already touched on some other key LDM deliverables and areas of responsibility, which are the Clinical Data Review Plan, the DMP, and the critical milestone of Clinical Database lock. Successful implementation and delivery of these items require LDMs to ensure for the Clinical Data Review Plan, sometimes also referred to as "Data Validation Plan (DVP)" or "Integrated Data Review Plan (IDRP)" to be in place and agreed upon cross-functionally to be the objective reference for evaluating, if data can be considered "reviewed" and ready for analysis, or not. There must not be alternative reviews by other functions that are documented properly in the Data Review Plan. If data review activities are shared between organizations such as a CRO and a sponsor company, it is imperative to work according to the same agreed-upon plan.

The key document of reference for all CDM-related activities is the DMP. The LDM makes sure that an initial version is in place before study-start and that any required updates, for this living document, are incorporated contemporaneously in such a way that the final DMP can be signed off before database lock, and serve as main documentation reference for regulatory audits or any other need to demonstrate how the study was executed from CDM's point of view.

All eyes will be on the LDM and the overall CDM team as database lock approaches. Tensions can rise easily, and it is a critical time for the LDM to firmly keep the hand on the rudder and steer the team through those anxious weeks and months toward database lock.

The Database Designer

Moving on to another lead role within CDM, we will have a look at the *(Clinical) Database Designer (DD)*. Similar to the LDM role, there are also different interpretations of this role throughout the industry. It can range from one end being a purely technical, more behind the scenes, role that focuses only on the design and programming of an EDC database, up to the other end of the spectrum, when the DD does not just look at the EDC environment, but leads and represents the implementation of all DCIs required for a given study. For the latter case the role names observed can be closer to "Clinical System Lead (CSL)" or similar and can refer to the approach when CDM takes accountability of all DCIs and therefore provides subject matter expertise on how all clinical data should be collected.

It goes back to the task of providing input to the clinical protocol and for the CSL, in this more advanced and broader interpretation of the role, to work with clinical teams and explore how technology could be deployed meaningfully to, for example, reduce the number of on-site visits for patients and therefore reduce their overall burden to participate in a clinical study. The decision for which medium should be used to collect clinical data is not a clinical one but should be driven by CDM with supportive input from other functions. Ideally the CSL, in collaboration with the LDM, can suggest to the team an overall clinical data flow for all data referenced in the clinical protocol, in such a way that the journey from true data source to final destination is clearly defined. A graphical representation of this flow is usually helpful and can easily be integrated as a part of the overall documentation in the DMP (see Figure 1.2).

I have seen CSLs also embracing the task to define data transfer specifications (DTS) for data originating from sources that do not require the design of new entry forms or the need to program/build a new database, for example data that is being sent from a central laboratory, where patients' blood samples have been analyzed. Even though this does not involve a typical programming approach, the combination of the LDM and CSL skill set is ideally suited to ensure that the area, which the industry often referred to as "external data handling", is taken care of adequately. Same as for other examples, I am not suggesting that CDM representatives should go solo on this task. Input from colleagues representing medical review, laboratory experts, and statistical programmers are also contributors to reducing the risk external data sets in general pose toward achieving a high-quality database lock on time.

In contrast to the LDM role, there is more fluctuation when it comes to the resource assignment of the DD throughout the study. CDM in general will have peak resources assignments across all roles in the months leading up to FPI, at interim database snapshots, before final database lock, and during mid-study changes, for example due to clinical protocol amendments. For the DD specifically though the peak assignment is during the original build

Clinical Data Flow for Study XXX1234

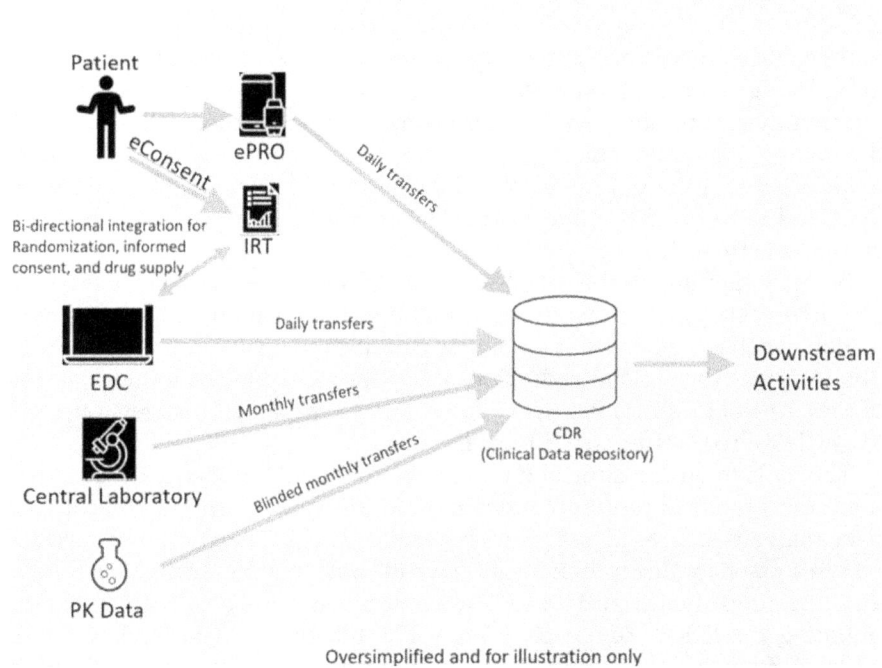

Oversimplified and for illustration only

FIGURE 1.2
Clinical Data Flow Illustration.

and set-up tasks before all DCIs go live, ideally before FPI. Assignments will extend into the early months of the ongoing study to address any required fixes or release remaining database components, which were not ready in time for a "Full Release" and therefore result in what is commonly known as a "Split Release". During the conduct phase of a clinical study the assignment can then go down to just a few hours per week to conduct periodic checks, update documentation requirements, and address any required fixes. It is beneficial to keep the DD assigned throughout the study, even with fewer hours, especially in larger CRO settings, where the mandate to maximize resource utilization might sometimes overwrite common sense approaches that would ensure continuity and clear accountability for these roles.

Let us illustrate it with a short example. Mistakes happen in database set-ups and the related programming all the time. Most of them will be identified and fixed through extensive validation procedures and user acceptance testing prior to going live. However, the post-production changes that will happen due to error fixes or mid-study changes are significantly more efficiently resolved by the DD who implemented them in the first place. If the original DD has been assigned to other activities and is not available anymore to address the tasks at hand, a new DD needs to be identified to either fix or change the database and/or programming for which that DD will not have any historic knowledge or reference. Readers with a programming background and experience will easily understand the reservations programmers typically have to inherit work from one of their colleagues. For the non-programmers among us, you can compare to getting a ¾ finished work of art and the task to finish it in the same style, color scheme, use of light, and same brushes, all of which might not be your personal preferences or areas of strength.

Before wrapping up the role description of the DD, as well as the broader CSL interpretation of it, we have to mention the creation of the tools that actually enable the clinical data review activities that we have already mentioned during the LDM introduction, and at the same time introduce the role of the Clinical Programmer (CP), who at some companies also gets referred to as CDM-Programmer or Clinical Developer.

The tools to enable clinical data review are mostly edit checks, data listings, and graphical representations of data to support, among other items, data analytics and trend analysis. This area of CDM is one of the best examples to show how the different roles have to come together to create a robust and meaningful clinical data review environment. It starts with the LDM initiating the IDRP (Remember? Yes – The Integrated Data Review Plan), which is my personal favorite description for the reference used to describe the Clinical Data Review Documentation. So, the LDM will facilitate the gathering of all(!) clinical data review requirements and document them in the IDRP, at which point either the DD or clinical programmer (CP), depending on skill set, experience, or process at a given company, will convert them into specifications that will be the foundation for the actual programming checks, listings, and graphs. The CP then performs the actual programming of the edit checks within the EDC system, as well as the listings and graphs in the environments of choice of the respective company.

The Tester

This is a good opportunity to introduce the role of the "Tester", for which there are also different company-specific role names. A few examples I came across are "Clinical Validation Analyst", "Clinical System Tester", or other variations thereof. For the purpose of this book and to hopefully reduce confusion, I am going to stick with "Tester", without meaning any disrespect for the important role and safeguard these individuals' play within clinical research.

Testers are a critical part of CDM fulfilling the step of an independent reviewer to test and validate that the outputs created through programming or system design activities match the previously agreed specifications. When we mentioned the importance of continuity within CDM roles and their assignments, testers can be seen a little bit as an outlier to this approach. Due to the importance of having an objective, neutral, and almost robotic approach to reviewing outputs and the underlying specifications, it is beneficial that they look at their tasks with fresh eyes every single time, rather than being assigned to the same programmer, client, or environment constantly.

One challenge with the tester role, and sometimes with CPs or programmers in general as well, that I have observed is the role interpretation by the individual or role implementation by the company being too narrow in scope and impact. Yes, the primary task for the tester is to ensure the program does what the specifications say. However, testers being the first line of defense could raise a flag, when obvious mistakes are encountered.

Let us look at an example for mistakes that can be detected early on by testers. If the specifications are asking to create an automated query in the EDC system, if the systolic blood pressure is greater than 1,600 mmHG, which would be an obvious typographical error in the specification, with the intended threshold being 160 mmHG. The CP then following the specifications, without questioning the obvious mistake and programming the edit check accordingly, and the tester later just validating that the edit check indeed raises a query for values larger than 1,600 and does not raise a query for a value like 1500, which would not be compatible with life, can, and probably should, flag the obvious typo in the specifications.

Some might say that CDM professionals do not necessarily have the background to be familiar with all the normal ranges used, like in this case for vital signs, or for other clinical data, which can be true for entry-level roles or for people just having entered the industry from a different field. The point that I want to make with this example is that regardless of the role or level or degree somebody has within CDM, and for that matter in Clinical Research in general, we need everybody to think about the broader impact their work has within the much bigger picture of conducting a clinical project. The reality in many companies though is that hierarchical structures, regional and cultural norms, and too narrowly and detailed worded Standard Operating Procedures (SOPs) are not conducive to invite people to speak up and challenge the "This is what we have always done" mentality.

The Clinical Data Coordinator

One of the most prominent roles in terms of headcount within CDM teams or serving as an entry point into the world of CDM is the *Clinical Data Coordinator (CDC)*. In terms of naming for this role, I have not seen too many variations to CDC, other than "Clinical Data Analyst", "Clinical Data Associate", or simply "Clinical Data Manager" as a catch-all. In terms of the role of the CDC, the main area of responsibility coming to mind, when I think about the CDC role, is to perform the data review tasks assigned to CDM. Concretely, it means to ensure that the queries raised by the automated edit checks within the EDC system are being addressed properly by the clinical site personnel. This includes checking the answers provided by the site and evaluating if the query can be closed or needs to be re-issued. This task requires a certain level of proficiency to navigate within EDC systems, which provides a hint toward the typical skill set and background professionals have, when they consider starting a career in CDM by starting as an entry-level CDC. An aptitude toward dealing with data, finding mistakes or patterns in abstract structures, and not adverse to the use of technology are common traits of people I have observed being successful and satisfied in the role of a CDC. It does not mean that people interested in the CDC role require a degree in computer science, nursing, pharmacy, or mathematics. In fact, there are countless examples of people becoming very successful CDCs (or other CDM entry-level roles such as Clinical Programmers) and propelling their career to more senior roles, without any of those scientific backgrounds.

Outside of the work done within the EDC system by CDCs, there is data review happening through clinical data listings or analytical tools in a separate environment. Typical examples are all sorts of reconciliation efforts when data from two different sources, such as EDC data and laboratory data, are being looked at to ensure that one source does not contradict the other.

However, bearing in mind that a typical career path within CDM toward the lead roles, such as the LDM, starts with expanding one's oversight, reach, and interpretation of the CDC role, it is common for CDCs with more years of experience to work hand in hand with the LDM. Reviewing the DMP, performing user acceptance testing (UAT), and updating the IDRP are just a few examples of how CDCs can assist the LDM and, at the same time, gain the required experience to eventually move on to a CDM Lead Role. It is worthwhile mentioning that some CDCs I have met throughout my professional journey are perfectly content to make this role their main career choice, without any ambition to move into an LDM role. When talking to these extraordinary experienced CDCs that might have decades of experience in this role, which often surpasses the experience levels of an LDM on a study they are assigned to, the most prominent reason they share for their decision to stay put is their enjoyment of staying close to the clinical data and the actions around it. They fully understand that lead and more senior roles come with a heavier load of administrative tasks and the need for periodic presentations for different stakeholders. The same way CDCs like to "keep their hands dirty" and stay close to the action, many CPs just enjoy the actual task of programming, without any desire to trade this in for managerial roles or any other lead assignments. I have the highest respect for these professionals who have found their sweet spot in the industry and provide such a significant, yet often hidden and underrecognized, contribution to the ultimate goal of a robust clinical data set. Especially larger corporations, both on the CRO and sponsor side, have accelerated the push to replace these experienced resources with lower cost options, not realizing that the reduced cost these companies think they can claim – at least on paper – increases the probability for costly re-work, quality issues, and loss of revenue due to customer dissatisfaction.

Other CDM Roles (Clinical Coders, SDTM Programmers, Clinical Data Scientists)

There are more roles associated with CDM, which are not consistently part of CDM departments across the industry. These include the roles of CCs, SDTM Programmers, and Clinical Data Scientists (CDSs).

Clinical Coders

Starting with the CCs, we are talking about a highly specialized role, with individuals who often do have medical degrees or a clinical or pharmacy background, without this having to be a knock-out criterion to become a CC. There are also examples of CDCs being able to be trained accordingly and take on CC responsibilities, without a degree or background in the afore-mentioned disciplines. The main responsibility for CCs consists in assigning a dictionary code for medications and diseases descriptions collected on the respective case report forms. This information is collected, for the most part, as free text on these forms and needs to be categorized and grouped in order to make it usable for data review and analysis later on. The standard coding dictionaries globally accepted and used throughout the industry are the "Medical Dictionary for Regulatory Activities" usually referred to as "MedDRA" for coding of diseases, and the WHODrug dictionary for the coding of any medicinal product.

To understand the complexity of the main CC task it is worthwhile to mention that in the latest MedDRA version there are more than 78,000 unique terms for the disease descriptions and more than half a million terms in the latest WHODrug dictionary for all the different medical products and variations thereof. CCs use medical coding tools, some of them with enhanced algorithms through the use of ML, to match the free text entered to describe the medical condition or medicinal product and assign the corresponding code from the dictionary to it. Even though some of the more advanced coding tools in the industry can reach high accuracy levels with auto code algorithms, the expertise provided by the human CC to ensure consistency within a given study and across an entire portfolio of studies for an investigational product is not replaceable at this point in time.

An additional complexity for the CCs to cope with is the periodic up-versioning of both dictionaries. Medical terms get fine-tuned and reclassified on an ongoing basis and new medical products being approved trigger the need to keep an eye on the latest versions available. As CCs are an important part of the overall data review approach, I believe that having Clinical Coding as a part of the CDM Team is the most logical approach. However, I have also seen Clinical Coding being embedded into the Pharmacovigilance group or being closely aligned with the Medical Monitoring Team. All these set-ups can work, as long as data review efforts do not become disjointed and are orchestrated in their entirety by the LDM.

The SDTM Programmer

While moving on to a role on the fringes of CDM – The SDTM Programmer – let's start with a short level-setting on Data Standards terminology. The Study Data Tabulation Model (SDTM) has become the de facto Data Standards used for clinical data, especially after the FDA had issued the requirement to submit data in SDTM for all studies that had started after December 17, 2016. SDTM is one of the data standards developed by the "Clinical Data Interchange Standards Consortium", or CDISC. The other two main data models used within Clinical Research, which were also developed by CDISC, are Clinical Data Acquisition Standards Harmonization (CDASH) and the Analysis Dataset Model (ADaM). As a short sidenote and not so serious warning, if you want to start a written communication with a hardcore Statistical Programmer on the wrong foot, just capitalize the "a" in "ADaM" – and see what happens.

The high-level takeaway about these Data Standards models from CDISC are that CDASH, as the name suggests, describes the metadata model during the data collection set-up for all DCIs, whereas SDTM is the data model used to organize, group, and structure data, after it has been collected. In addition, transforming clinical data into SDTM allows for more seamless integration between different parties, running data analytics tools in a more standardized approach and ensuring compliance with regulatory requirements for data submissions. Lastly, ADaM is being used as the foundation to run the actual analysis of a clinical study, by facilitating the grouping of clinical data, and the derivation of new data, according to the Statistical Analysis Plan (SAP).

Looking at the SDTM Programmer role within the industry there are CDM teams that see the conversion of raw or CDASH data into SDTM data as a CDM delivery and therefore the SDTM Programmer sitting within the CDM department. On the other hand, you see the more prominent approach in the industry where Statistical Programmers, as part of the Biostatistics and Programming Team, perform the SDTM programming task.

Having seen both approaches firsthand and keeping in mind the benefit of avoiding roles with a very narrow area of responsibility, I prefer and recommend keeping the end-to-end programming tasks pertaining to SDTM conversion, ADaM dataset preparation, and the culmination with the creation of the Tables Listings and Figures (TLFs) for analysis, with the Statistical Programming Team outside of CDM. The main reasons being to avoid an unnecessary handover between two teams when it comes to transitioning from SDTM to ADaM, and to allow more senior Statistical Programmers to engage in the full spectrum of Statistical Programming.

The Clinical Data Scientist

With the increase of Data Analytics capabilities and the regulatory framework not only allowing but strongly encouraging risk-based approaches when it comes to clinical study oversight, the role of the *Clinical Data Scientist (CDS)* has become increasingly popular within the industry.

The best way that I have come across so far to describe the Data Analytics tasks CDSs perform is to imagine a clinical study and its data as a huge forest with the trees representing the patients in the study and the leaves being the individual data points. Many CDSs would argue that their CDC counterparts in CDM look at the individual leaves or maybe a branch to ensure those data points are logical, and that medical review might look at an entire tree (representing all data for one patient) through patient profile review. CDSs, however, fly with drones over the entire forest to identify areas where a group of trees look different from others and look for anything that could be a worrisome trend, which can only be seen from the sky, but not while looking at individual trees or leaves. I really like this analogy as it illustrates key aspects of clinical data review in general. However, does the fact that one group has to climb on trees, while the other can fly drones over them – begging your pardon by surely stretching the analogy a little too far – justify a departmental separation, when the goal for both teams is the same?

It is interesting to observe that in some companies the CDS role is fully integrated within the CDM department, whereas in other places it is either its own department or part of Clinical Operations. It is an ongoing topic of discussion, and I find it fascinating how passionately the proponents of keeping CDS separate from CDM argue their case. Yes, the exploratory analyses, statistical considerations, trend identifications, and possibly broader clinical background many CDSs bring to the table do make them a very unique and valuable asset in every company. Nonetheless, to avoid further fragmentation of the data review process across even more departments, which triggers the need for more documentation and handovers and increasing the risk of either duplicating review efforts or leaving gaps while assuming somebody else might take care of a certain review, I have seen more cohesive and reliable data review performances, when the CDS mindset and role is fully integrated within the CDM team. In addition, there is a clear career path from CDC to CDS while embracing the full spectrum of clinical data for analytical purposes.

(Clinical) Data Entry Specialist

For more than a decade now, I have not come across any CDM personnel working as (Clinical) Data Entry Specialists anymore, which is not surprising as the paper-CRF days are surely behind us. Nonetheless, maybe more for nostalgic reasons, I am feeling obliged to at least mention this once vital role in CDM, which for some of today's CDM Department Heads was how they started in the industry. The occasional paper record still finds its way into the data flow in some studies. In these cases, due to the nonexistent DEs,

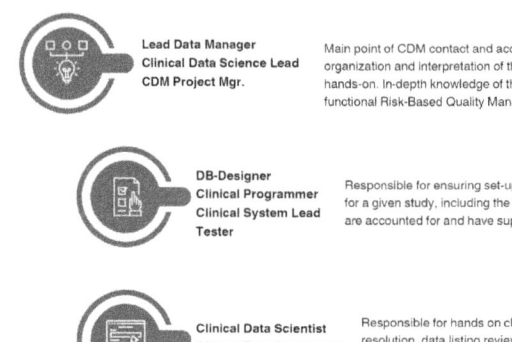

Lead Data Manager
Clinical Data Science Lead
CDM Project Mgr.
Main point of CDM contact and accountable for overall study-related items. Depending on the organization and interpretation of the role, it can be more Project Management oriented or more hands-on. In-depth knowledge of the study is required for either scenario. Ideally leading cross-functional Risk-Based Quality Management (RBQM)

DB-Designer
Clinical Programmer
Clinical System Lead
Tester
Responsible for ensuring set-up and validation of the ideal system landscape and clinical data flow for a given study, including the set-up of any data review tools. Ensuring that all clinical data sources are accounted for and have supporting documentation in place

Clinical Data Scientist
Clinical Data Coordinator
Responsible for hands on clinical data review, including, but not limited to, automated edit check resolution, data listing reviews, data science driven exploratory reviews, trend analysis, overall support and input for RBQM

Clinical Coder
(SDTM Programmer)
Clinical Coders fulfil a key role toward clinical data quality by ensuring consistent grouping of medical terms and medications using industrywide accepted terminology originating primarily from the MedDRA and WHODrug dictionaries. Their activity often includes reconciliation of codes between the clinical and the Pharmacovigilance databases. SDTM Programmers are more often found under the umbrella of Statistical Programming

FIGURE 1.3
Overview of CDM Roles and Responsibilities.

a common approach is to assign junior-level CDCs or some trained administrative staff to complete these tasks.

In Figure 1.3, I wrap up the CDM role overview and the acknowledgement that there are likely other role names and interpretations used in companies throughout the industry.

More important though, than the naming of a role and defining its area of responsibilities through SOPs, is the understanding of the full spectrum of tasks that CDM Professionals should lead or at least be involved in, regardless of the name that is assigned to it.

When the profession of CDM emerged in the early 1990s, it was not uncommon that just one person, typically with some sort of technical background, would cover most, if not all, of the tasks described earlier. This was before CDISC Standards existed or 21 CFR Part 11 was published by the FDA. This one "Tech"-Person, as official role names for CDM were not common yet, would set up a clinical database for manual double data entry, which often was based on homegrown technology. They would support the creation of a three-part-NCR (stands for "No Carbon Required", maybe an idea for a nice trivia question at your next CDM department meeting) Case Report Form (CRF), program some basic edit checks and listings for data review, create so-called Data Clarification Forms (DCFs) to be sent or faxed to clinical sites, and possibly assist the biostatistics team with the analysis of study results. And guess what? New medicinal products got approved by regulatory agencies and were released to the public as well.

In summary, one commonality of successful CDM departments that I have observed over the last three decades, and the positive impact it has on the overall company, is the mindset of not only accepting the accountability when offered, but determinedly pursuing it when not in CDM hands, for all clinical-data-related tasks, looking at every CDM role, not in isolation and in a head-down approach, but in a CDM Team approach, where we have specialists for certain areas who understand and identify with the goal of the Team, that is, the delivery of reliable data.

Being a CDM professional can be a very rewarding and fulfilling career choice with phenomenal growth opportunities, if the company's environment and culture paired with one's willingness to embrace accountability exist.

CDM Deliverables

Now that we have established the framework and reason for Clinical Data's unique value within Clinical Research and defined the most prominent roles within CDM, we will move on by diving into the deliverables that CDM should embrace, lead, and take accountability for.

Looking at it from the highest possible level, the mission statement for CDM is straight forward – "Deliver high-quality clinical data which is fit for purpose". The purpose is to support the planned analysis according to the SAP and therefore to answer questions about safety and efficacy for the investigational product. What does "high quality" mean? One way to answer the question is to point to the broadly accepted principles of ALCOA (Attributable, Legible, Contemporaneous, Original, Accurate) or ALCOA++ (ALCOA plus Complete, Consistent, Enduring and Available). In addition to the ALCOA approach, something that I have found very helpful throughout my career is to ask:

1. How can I ensure through CDM excellence that the final clinical data reflects reality?
2. Can I firmly stand behind every process step that collects, touches, changes, im- or exports, derives, and reports clinical data, and explain it thoroughly and with confidence in a regulatory audit situation?

Using the schematic below as a reference of CDM scope, we will analyze the following deliverables and the criteria that will ensure regulatory compliance and reliable results to achieve them:

- Data Management Plan (DMP)
- Database Design (Using EDC as an example)
- Clinical Data Review and Integrated Data Review Plan (IDRP)
- Database Lock

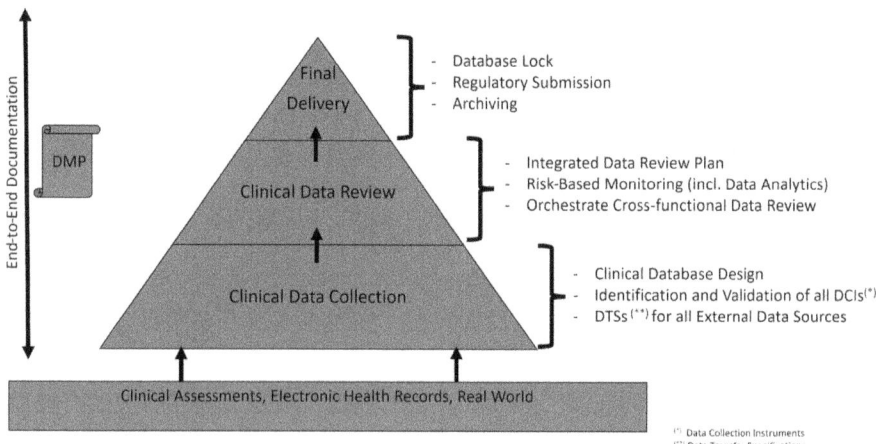

FIGURE 1.4
Overview of CDM Delivery.

We can easily see the flow and dependencies of CDM deliverables in Figure 1.3. The clinical data that has been defined in the protocol and that we are after is out there. Out there in clinical assessments that still need to happen, out there in already existing medical records, and out there in the real world waiting to be collected. After and during collection the focus is on Review and then the preparation for analysis. All of which is documented in the data management plan (DMP). So, let's start with the DMP.

The Data Management Plan

The DMP is the key reference document for all CDM activities – no exception! I can almost hear the outcry from some of you about the "no exception" part and thinking about items such as specification documents, clinical coding guidelines as a stand-alone document, or CDM project management activities. How can all this fit into one DMP, without creating a monstrous and unmanageable nightmare document?

Having faced this question frequently and understanding the valid concerns fueling it, I do like to remind the skeptics of the alternative to the centralized DMP. Following the regulatory requirements in our industry, all activities need to be documented and the standard processes, or required deviations thereof, clearly identified. The alternative to a centralized DMP would mean that the person who has to tell the CDM story for a given study or overall submission, in most cases the LDM and/or CDM Leadership, would have to find all the scattered documentation-puzzle pieces and put them together in a cohesive summary. So why not start with a centralized DMP in the first place? The centralization and unambiguous mandate to have all CDM activities for a given study in one DMP is not the only success factor to ensure audit readiness and an organized approach for CDM. Even more important is the use of a DMP Template that contains all the distinct, yet connected, CDM tasks in dedicated chapters within the document. The Society for Clinical Data Management (SCDM; www.scdm.org), which I will reference a few times throughout this book, has a clear overview and example of chapters that should be part of a DMP (https://scdm.org/gcdmp/). In my experience, having used this approach in a good number of audits, I suggest the following chapters as a starting point:

- CDM Personnel
- Communication & Oversight
- Database Design (EDC)
- External Data (Identification & Handling)
- Clinical Data Flow Chart
- Data Review (Including Data Analytics and items such as Quality Tolerance Limits [QTLs]) and a reference to the Integrated Data Review Plan (IDRP)
- Clinical Coding
- CDM Project Management
- Metrics
- Database Lock and Unlock
- SOPs used (including deviations or notes to file)
- Archiving and decommission.

There are subcategories such as System Validation and Testing that can be its own chapter or referenced in the existing Database Design Chapter. The same is true for "System Access Management". Depending on the company and preferences, topics such as "Serious Adverse Events Handling and Reconciliation" can be a chapter on its own or addressed under "Data Review".

The key differentiator though, which ultimately will drive adherence and compliance of the centralized use of DMPs is . . . Drumroll Please . . . to structure and write the chapters in such a way that they refer to the standard processes, guidelines, and templates that are in place within the CDM department.

This results in most chapters starting with the yes/no question "Did this study <X> follow the standard process <Y> to achieve outcome <Z> (Yes/No)?"

If the answer is "Yes" then the main part of the documentation is done; however, if the answer is "No" then the LDM or designated DMP author will have to:

- justify why there has been a deviation from the standard approach and
- describe which process was implemented for this study.

The positive results of this proven approach are manifold. It starts with much higher adherence rates to established standard processes within the department. On the flipside it is also very telling when the number of required and documented deviations in DMPs increases, which is then a possible indicator that the standard processes in place might be outdated and should be considered for a review.

Additional benefit from a templated DMP, which is based on checking if a given study followed the standard approaches or not, is that DMP reviews by managerial staff and/or Quality Assurance (QA) representatives are much more efficient, because the amount of free language and long narratives is reduced. Furthermore, the "Yes"-answered chapters only need to be checked to be truly adhering to the standard processes, while the "No"-answered chapters will need a more in-depth review.

In 2007, I ventured to share the benefits of such a DMP implementation with my industry peers during the annual SCDM conference, which was in Chicago that year. The slightly provocative title of my presentation was "How to create a DMP in One Day". I recall starting the talk with the question "How many of you believe that you can create the starting version of a DMP in just one day?" Exactly one hand out of the approximately 300 attendees went up (Thank you, Dan Miller, for believing me early on ☺).

However, when I had gone through the structure, reasoning, and the actual benefits of the templated and standardized DMP approach and was about to conclude my presentation, I did ask the audience the same question again and was pleased to see that Dan was not alone with his opinion anymore.

Now, almost two decades later, standardized DMP approaches have become more the norm and the resulting gains in efficiency and usability are now even more needed than before, due to the increases in study complexity, and volume and variety of data sources.

To check if the DMP approach in your company is adequate, simply ask yourself if you could answer any CDM-related question from an auditor for a given study during an inspection, by referencing first a chapter in the corresponding DMP. You will be able to approach an audit situation much more confidently if you can address the most popular questions from auditors around System access, External Data Set Processing, Data Review Activities, Database Lock and Unlock Procedures, Process Deviations, and so on. By referencing the DMP and consistently starting your answers with "In Chapter X of our DMP we have documented the deployed process and have references to all the supporting documents, forms and signatures", auditors will realize the organized approach your organization has implemented to document all CDM-related activities.

Figure 1.5 depicts the DMP Pyramid showing the Clinical Study as a basis and how the DMP is the go-to, tip of the iceberg, entry point for all CDM documentation for this study. This image was used by me during an information session at the FDA with auditor trainees in attendance.

CDM Best Practices

The DMP (Data Management Plan) Pyramid

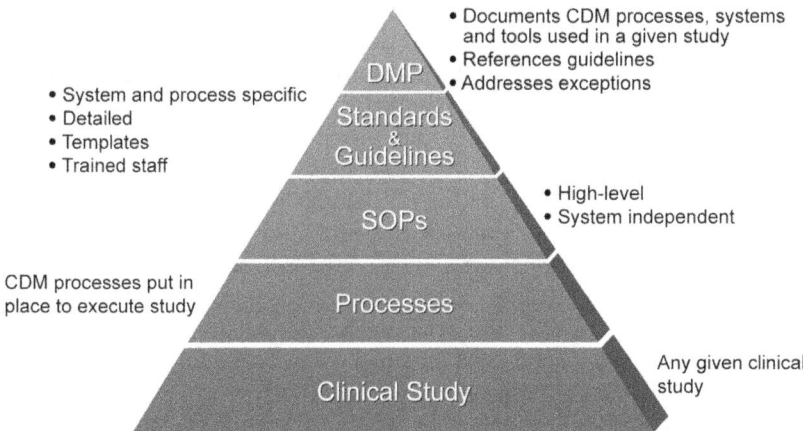

• System and process specific
• Detailed
• Templates
• Trained staff

CDM processes put in place to execute study

DMP

Standards & Guidelines

SOPs

Processes

Clinical Study

• Documents CDM processes, systems and tools used in a given study
• References guidelines
• Addresses exceptions

• High-level
• System independent

Any given clinical study

FIGURE 1.5
The DMP Pyramid.

Database Design

We have already established that clinical data is at the heart of Clinical Research. One important aspect of clinical data is how to collect it. Even though from a pure volume perspective the amount of data coming from non-EDC sources is usually much larger, EDC still is and will be for the foreseeable future a significant component of clinical data collection and aggregation. Therefore, the design of the EDC database, integrations between EDC and other data sources such as Randomization and Trial Supply Management (RTSM) data, and the set-up of any other DCI deemed necessary for the clinical study at hand are other pivotal CDM-led deliverables.

The LDM working hand in hand with the DD, or similar role such as the CSL, determines, based on the protocol requirements, which clinical data is best suited to be collected via EDC and explores opportunities for other collection methods, if there can be quality and/or efficiency gains by getting closer to source data. Concretely, this means to evaluate whether direct access to electronic health records (EHR) is a feasible option for upcoming studies.

Lessening the burden for participating patients by considering ePRO technology and direct patient outreach through home-health nurses collecting required study data are additional items that will influence the final DCI Landscape. The guiding principle for the CDM Team leading the DCI

landscape design and aligning with the requirements from other departments, such as Clinical Operations, is to focus on keeping it as streamlined
and simple as possible, reduce the number of integrations and people having
to "touch" the data, as well as shorten the distance between the true data
source and its final destination. As an example, it used to be considered best-
practice in the early EDC dates, to load Central Laboratory data into the EDC
environment. The main driver behind this approach was the desire, and possibly more comfortable feeling, to have all data in one place. Especially at the
time of database lock, it seemed to facilitate the proof that no data had been
changed after locking the database and removing all required access rights
to it. Even though the goal of having all data eventually in one place is laud-
able, it did not justify the burden behind repeated uploading of the Central
Laboratory data, which represents the largest dataset in most studies, and
having to decide between either incremental loads and the complicated logic
behind them to ensure only the new or changed data gets added, or to go
with cumulative loads and deal with audit trail overflows or runtime errors,
because of the immense volume. CDM eventually realized that there was
no gain for this "Detour" for the Central Laboratory Data to be loaded into
EDC only to be extracted again after database lock and then for analysis
later on. Other arguments around trying to advocate for Central Laboratory
data loads into EDC were pointing to the need for the Principal Investigators
(PIs) at the clinical sites to have access to this data for their clinical evaluation. This argument became obsolete, when PIs were able to access this data
directly and timely, by accessing data visualizations offered by those providers of non-EDC data.

Therefore, as a CDM professional involved or accountable for the design
of DCIs, every suggested integration should be questioned for its supposed
value added. Especially when dealing with technology vendors for any sort
of DCIs used in a clinical study, be it an EDC, ePRO, eConsent, RTSM, or
specialty laboratory, it is crucially important for CDM to not get bamboozled
by all the shiny technical possibilities offered, but to decide for the most
pragmatic and efficient solution possible to satisfy the specific study needs.
Just because an integration is "possible" and can be "seamless", "automated",
or as recently heard "artificially 'intelligenced'", all adjectives used by some
technology representatives, does not mean that CDM should give the green
light for it.

Using EDC as an example to look at the actual design process, which is
applicable for other DCIs as well, is to evaluate the extent to which existing Standards can facilitate the build process and increase quality at the
same time. Being able to use previously validated and accepted data entry
forms, underlying metadata and related automated edit checks, is a huge
advantage. If you work at a company with an established Data Standards
Team, or at least CDM personnel assigned to create and maintain CDISC
based Standards, you are in a very fortunate position and should take full
advantage of it. If, on the flipside, your work environment did not allow yet

to invest into the creation of a Data Standards Library, or such a Library does exist, but is constantly overwritten by individual preferences, I do recommend to make it a departmental goal to create a role or team of Data Standards Stewarts who will build and, within reason, enforce the use of these standards through increased cross-functional dialogue. For smaller companies with a limited number of studies, and therefore reduced benefit of investing in Data Standards, the engagement with CDM service providers who offer established Data Standards can be beneficial.

Regardless of whether a Program-First or Specification-First approach is the preference, the database design process needs to include validation procedures to ensure that either the resulting EDC system, as an example, satisfies the requirements provided through the specifications, or the specifications created by the system after implementation address all the requirements. In addition to the more programming-oriented validation, UAT by people in roles representing the real-life users of the EDC system will reduce the error rate and the need for avoidable post-production changes.

Before wrapping up the Database Design Deliverable, I feel compelled to address one myth around the time, sometimes referred to as cycle time, it takes, or should take, to create a fully functional EDC database with all its data entry forms, automated edit checks, required integrations, CRF Completion Guidelines (CCGs), clinical coding environments, and other ancillary items. This must be one of the most prominent, yet in my opinion irrelevant question, I have been asked during vendor evaluation meetings or within the same company from colleagues outside of CDM: "Michael, how long does it take your team to build an EDC database?" If the interrogator wanted to make an even stronger argument, or pretend to have some expertise in this area, the question would be extended by something like: ". . . just to let you know, your competitor said they can do it in less than 8 weeks . . .". The actual issue that matters in this context is not how long it takes to build the full database, but to ensure it goes live before FPI, as otherwise it could put timely data entry and review of the early assessments in jeopardy. Database design activities typically start with a robust Clinical Protocol Synopsis. Bearing in mind that the time between the finalized Clinical Protocol and FPI is very rarely less than 12 weeks, an appropriately resourced CDM team can easily build a high-quality database with all its required components before FPI, especially if established data standards can be used for part of the database development. Risks to achieve this goal can emerge by factors outside of CDM, for example when last minute protocol amendments happen, which alter visit schedules or the clinical data that had been targeted originally.

Thus, the take-home message related to the CDM database development cycle-time from stable/final clinical protocol to go-live of EDC does not have a certain number of weeks as the correct answer. Service providers claiming they can do it in 2 weeks are likely referring to a very basic clinical study with a reduced number of unique forms and most of the database components being copied from a "sister study". More importantly though, the point being missed by these service providers is that even if this EDC database can be released in 2 weeks, what is the benefit of then having this database sitting idle for 10+ weeks while waiting for FPI to happen? It only increases the risk of protocol changes to happen during that time, which will trigger re-work that could have been avoided by targeting a final database go-live date about a week before the planned FPI date and therefore leaving some buffer to fix possible last-minute issues.

The quickest EDC Database development for a full go-live with all the required integrations and data review tools needed that I have ever witnessed was 5 weeks. The only reason why my team pushed for such an aggressive goal was that FPI actually had a realistic chance to happen for this COVID trial, for which the clinical protocol was finished very quickly, and the reduced number of clinical sites planned for it had already been used for previous studies and were able to complete the required regulatory tasks in a matter of weeks.

Clinical Data Review and Integrated Data Review Plan (IDRP)

Next, we are going to discuss what is arguably the core and most challenging activity for CDM – Clinical Data Review, colloquially also referred to as "Data Cleaning".

Starting again with the nomenclature associated with this deliverable there are reasons to stay away from the word "clean" when referring to clinical data deemed ready for analysis, or in the context of a "Clean Patient" when referring to the clinical data pertaining to one particular patient being fully reviewed. In my opinion, the word "clean" in the context of CDM carries some subjectivity of what individuals, teams, or entire companies have in mind, when describing the quality and readiness of clinical data. Experienced CDM professionals know that there is no such thing as a "clean" database or "clean" subject, because every time a database is considered "clean", a modified or more expansive data review approach will always find additional items for a dataset to be then considered "dirty", to stay within the same vocabulary bubble.

Therefore, and to emphasize the guiding principles behind the Clinical Data Review task, which are as follows:

- Objective
- Reproducible
- Systematic

I suggest referring to clinical data as "reviewed" or "not (fully) reviewed" according to a predefined IDRP.

This approach immediately tackles the requirement of objectivity and reproducibility. Let us look at it more closely, starting with the center piece – the IDRP.

If I had to rank CDM items from most to least important to determine the likelihood of a successfully executed clinical study, the IDRP would take one of the top positions, if not the top one. To be unambiguously clear, CDM, in the person of the LDM or equivalent role, is accountable for the creation, maintenance, and executions of the IDRP, with cross-functional input and support. Concretely, the LDM must ensure that every role involved in data review activities provides input for the IDRP in such a way that every antici-pated review will be defined and documented in the IDRP. In other words, it should be made impossible to create a data query automatically by the system, or manually by any data reviewer, if the logic behind this query or the justification for the manual review that created this query has no corre-sponding reference, and therefore CDM approval, in the IDRP. This is how objectivity for clinical data review is achieved, as issuing a data query will not be based on the subjective view of a Medical Reviewer, the experience level of a CDC, the personal preference of a Statistical Programmer, or the possible incentive for a service provider to issue as many queries as possible as they might get paid by the number of queries issued.

The depth and extent of data review are also influenced by the planned statistical analysis defined in the SAP in terms of primary and secondary endpoints for the clinical study. Going back to the word "clean" and the prin-ciple of being *objective* when performing clinical data review, it should be apparent now that a cross-functionally approved IDRP becomes the objec-tive reference for a clinical study team to declare a patient or an entire study "Reviewed!".

Looking at the other two principles for clinical data review, that is, *Reproducible* and *Systematic*, I will share, as an example, a frequent dialogue I used to have with our colleagues in Medical Review, who often use a "Patient Profile" tool or graphical representation to see all clinical data for a specific patient at once. The Medical Reviewer's task is to ensure the data presented for this patient makes sense from a medical point of view.

I had many Medical Monitors admit that their review might be quite sub-jective for areas such as determining clinical significance of medical condi-tions and if they should constitute an AE or not. Furthermore, they conceded that two different Medical Reviewers might come to different conclusions and possibly issue queries or accept data as is. I fully appreciate the diffi-culty of the Medical Review task and acknowledge that there are gray areas that cannot be compared to the much simpler binary approaches for cer-tain edit checks, where values are either in a predetermined range or not. Nonetheless, with the important contribution of Medical Review and by extension, Exploratory Review in general, which by definition cannot be pre-defined, as the name itself suggests, that is, "exploratory", any possible data issues identified by this sort of review should be incorporated into the IDRP.

You might wonder how the unknown can be documented in the IDRP. Successful approaches that I have seen specify medical and exploratory review as part of the overall plan in the IDRP, and, very importantly, mention that any possible findings will be generalized and translated into study-wide systematic checks and automated if possible.

An example might be helpful to understand this approach. A typical laboratory normal range for Alanine Transaminase (ALT) is around 7–50 units per liter of blood. One Medical Reviewer looking at a Patient Profile summary with an ALT of 65 and taking other items such as Medical History, Age, and previous laboratory samples in considerations might feel inclined to query the site to check if an AE should be recorded, especially if the investigational product might come with some hepatic-related concerns from previous studies, whereas another Medical Reviewer might not be as concerned and be comfortable without sending a query. To ensure that in this specific example the IDRP gets updated appropriately and cohesive review of the entire Medical Review will take place afterward, the LDM should seek clarification from the Medical Team, if a targeted check can be put in place that flags all cases systematically of elevated ALTs (providing a specific value) and all other relevant factors that would trigger a query to follow up with the site to check for a possibly missed AE.

There must only be ONE IDRP per study, even if, or better said, especially when, multiple companies are involved in running a clinical study, for example, when a Biotech or Pharma company engages with a CRO to provide CDM and other services. Even though the danger of having multiple Review Plans in place, or having isolated teams performing detached, borderline clandestine, data review activities, should be obvious to any Clinical Research Professional, it continues to be mindboggling to me how often it is still happening throughout the industry. It is my hope that sharing with you some of the most prominent examples, unfortunately based on true stories, of fragmented clinical data review will help to shed some light on this calamity and reduce its occurrence going forward.

Example 1: Biotech Company Outsourcing CDM to a CRO

The CRO had a cross-functional IDRP in place; however, the Biotech Company insisted on implementing a "Sponsor Review", which the Biotech Company did not want to share with the CRO in terms of scope and extent. This approach is just wrong on so many levels. It puts the CRO in a losing position from the beginning as it is incredibly easy to find holes in an IDRP, if 2 teams with different agendas want to look at data. The Biotech company seemed more interested in proving the CRO CDM team wrong, than actually working together and having the common goal of getting to "Reviewed Data" as one team and serve the greater good in terms of running a successful clinical study. Having these disjoined review teams not sharing their individual review plans caused inefficiencies due to overlapping reviews and contradicting queries sent to the sites, as well as gaps due to the false assumptions that the other team might take care of certain reviews. Some of you might think that this particular Biotech company was just trying to fulfill their regulatory obligation to provide oversight of the outsourced activity. If that were the case, the correct approach should have been to participate, review, and approve the One IDRP from the CRO, and monitor the clinical data review progress through the type of queries issued and frequent communication with the data review team to see if updates to the One IDRP were needed. If the Biotech company had valid reasons for additional review activities by their specialized Medical Review Team, this review should have been documented and implemented in the same IDRP for overall transparency and avoidance of overlapping activity.

Example 2: Certain Functions Not Being Included in the IDRP

At some companies the accountability for declaring a subject "Reviewed" does not lie with CDM, but with other functional representatives or might even be undefined. These are the companies where CDM either has not embraced, or was not allowed to embrace, the full accountability for Data Review. In these places CDM is often limited to dealing with the automated queries in EDC and some basic data reconciliation tasks. These items are then documented in a basic Data Review Plan for CDM; however other review, and query generating, activities, by Medical Review, Clinical Operations, Pharmacovigilance, SDTM Programming, and so on get performed without the required objective, reproducible, and systematic foundation. When I had the opportunity to discuss with these clinical study teams their approach and asking them directly about how they were determining when a data was ready for database lock and analysis, some of the answers were even more shocking than the process itself. One of the most concerning answers I heard was that certain team members, excluding CDM, would vote, Yes Vote! to see if there was a majority thinking that data was "clean" enough to proceed. Even though I am huge proponent of democracy in general, clinical data review is not a place for democracy, but for the requirement of an all-encompassing and objective reference documenting which rules were followed to declare data "reviewed".

In summary for Clinical Data Review, the key items for CDM to remember is to embrace the accountability for the overall activity and lead the cross-functional, possibly cross-company, teams toward a unified, agreed-upon and approved IDRP. Look out for opportunities to reduce subjectivity and manual review activities that can be converted into automated edit checks or exception listings, facilitating the review and increasing consistency.

The IDRP itself, or a reference to it, should be part of the DMP, within the chapter dedicated to the documentation of data review.

Database Lock

The Database Lock is likely the most prominent of all CDM deliverables. The time – in some companies unfortunately the only time – when all eyes seem to be directed at CDM is when the planned Database Lock is only a few weeks away. Suddenly the entire study team redirected their focus toward CDM. Our colleagues outside of CDM will now start asking questions about outstanding queries, missing CRF pages, delayed external data set transfers and reconciliations, or clinical coding targets not being coded yet.

Throughout study conduct the LDM will surely have provided updates on the aforementioned parameters; however, mid-study the main areas of interest are usually patient enrollment and site performances. This changes as soon as the LPI milestone is achieved and when the Project Manager can determine the planned LPO date and target when the database should be locked. A more successful approach for the LDM, leading CDM activities for the overall study, and having the Database Lock milestone in mind from the beginning, even though it might be months or even years away, is to ensure that the periodic CDM updates in study team meetings are a standing agenda item and conducted in a way that they are meaningful for the other functions. As an example, it is not a good approach and a lost opportunity to use the CDM timeslot to just rattle off numbers for queries, missing pages, and similar items without context. LDMs should use the full power of data analytics and the recently released regulatory guidance for risk-based approaches to inform the study team throughout the entire length of the study, starting at Day 1, about what the incoming clinical data, and possibly metadata originating from audit trails, is telling us in terms of possible risks. Are there sites not entering data on time? Are we approaching certain predefined QTLs? Do we have CRAs performing SDR, but then this data changes again? Do we have data backlogs associated with certain sites or regions? The list goes on and on. The point is that when database lock is approaching these updates, the messages they carry should not come as a surprise for the team anymore. In fact, in some well-executed implementations of this approach, I have seen a healthy, almost sporty, kind of competition emerging from clinical sites, CRAs, and other teams to do their part throughout the study, not just at the end when threatened.

Even with the best preparation and fully supportive and collaborative teams, Database Locks are often demanding and will have some bumps until it is finally done. This should not come as a surprise as all the combined efforts and activities culminate in this one key milestone. All the different data sources must have delivered their final transfer; all team members deem the data as "Reviewed"; Biostatistics and Statistical Programming are getting ready to receive and unblind the locked data to run their analysis; all PIs from the sites must have signed and endorsed the data from their end; and all required documentations, such as the DMP, IDRP, and Database Lock Form, need the signatures to confirm their final status. With all these moving parts in place, and often at least one of them failing in the final steps toward Database lock, it is crucial for the LDM, representing the person orchestrating these final steps, to keep calm and in control. The eyes will be on the LDM to make the decision to possibly having to delay Database Lock by a day or two, if certain issues cannot be addressed in time and are too critical to be ignored, or on the flipside, to proceed with a Database Lock, because the remaining issues are of such a nature that it can be proven that they will not have an impact whatsoever on the analysis, or pose any risk, as minimal as it might be, to patient's safety.

CDM Driving Cross-functional Work and Excellence

I now wrap this chapter up with the goal of encouraging and empowering every CDM professional to fully embrace the role and accountability that comes with it in their respective company. Whether it is the LDM, CDSL, CSL, CDC, DD, Tester, CC, or other description used to define a CDM role, the matter of fact is that you, in your CDM role, are the ultimate subject matter expert (SME) for the area you cover. An LDM not taking the lead for the IDRP, a CSL not taking the lead for the overall system landscape, or a tester not flagging obvious mistakes in the specifications leave a void that will either increase the probability for data quality issues or force/invite other functional representatives to fill that void for CDM. During one of my CDM consultancy assignments, I was attending my very first meeting, which was titled "Data Review Meeting". It turned out to be a cross-functional meeting with the goal of looking at how data review activities were progressing for a pivotal study. Even though CDM was well represented in that meeting, it turned out that a Clinical Operations Representative was leading that meeting, as well as all other cross-functional data-focused meetings. When I asked about the set-up and why CDM was not coordinating these activities, it turned out that CDM had been an afterthought at that company from the very beginning, when there had not even been a CDM department. The role was diminished to a purely technical assignment. I should point out that the Clinical Operations representative stepping into this CDM void did relatively well in trying to do what the LDM should have been doing; however, it did result in cumbersome and not efficient review activities, in the form of countless excel trackers, using EDC functionality improperly to "stabilizing" data, focusing on meaningless metrics, and losing track of the actual bottlenecks of the study. I also found confirmation again that the task of reviewing data, seeing query counts balloon, and then trying to get that number back under control is a very rewarding and satisfying task, which different roles seem to gravitate to during certain periods of time, forgetting that there is actually a role that should be doing it throughout the study, which is the LDM. I want to tell those team members that, if you like to review clinical data that much, enjoy pattern detection, finding trends, wanting to ensure overall data quality, well, then become a CDM professional, as this might be your true calling.

Summary

We have taken the first step into the fascinating world of CDM by defining the most valuable asset that is being entrusted to us – Clinical Data. This created the question of "Who is 'us'?" which we answered by a detailed overview of the most prominent CDM roles. With these two main pillars in place, Clinical Data and the Custodians thereof, we ventured into exploring the tasks that result as a logical consequence from it.

It is my hope that you either already knew about the unique role of CDM and got corroborative evidence and examples for your point of view, or your CDM experience to date has been more of a supporting role and you start seeing the opportunities and responsibilities that are looming ahead for you.

In the next chapter we will venture even further into the data universe, almost literally, and see, think about, and possibly even feel clinical data as you might have never felt it before.

2

Dissecting Clinical Data to Its "Atomic" Structure. The Case for AI and ML in CDM

Here, we will approach and look at clinical data from a completely new perspective and in ways probably never done before. Along the way, we explore questions such as "How trustworthy is any clinical data point in our database?" or "Is source data the ultimate truth or can it also be wrong?" Part of the answers to these questions will include a personal story about unearthing actual fraud at a clinical site.

The goal for us is to further develop the "CDM mindset", which is similar to a sixth sense alerting us to any possible factor that could jeopardize the integrity of a data point.

We will also dive into the AI discussion, by starting with some number comparisons between possible data permutations in a typical clinical study and compare it to our universe. This, together with a closer look into the audit trail, will create the basis for actual examples of AI applications in our industry.

In this chapter, we will cover the following topics:

- Exploring the trustworthiness of clinical data
- Atoms in the universe
- The power of the audit trail
- The case for AI in CDM

Exploring the Trustworthiness of Clinical Data

Now that we have established the unique value of clinical data, introduced some of the key roles within CDM, and provided examples and arguments for CDM professionals to embrace the accountability to become the end-to-end custodians of this valuable asset, let us explore more in depth what we actually mean when we talk about "clinical data".

How accurate are the data points we collected and reviewed for a clinical assessment, such as an electrocardiogram (ECG)?

Are we getting the full picture and complete understanding of what the investigational product is doing to the patients in terms of benefits and/or possible harm?

These are just a few questions for which we will try to find the answers. Buckle up as we are now jumping headfirst into the Clinical Data Universe.

Almost all clinical data points follow a common description allowing them to be associated to a patient's assessment conducted at a given point in time according to the clinical protocol. Exceptions are items such as laboratory normal ranges which are not patient specific and require different identifiers, such as a laboratory identification number and codes for the descriptions of the laboratory parameters being used.

For the patient-related data, however, there always is a group of data points to identify either directly or implicitly the "Who?" "What?" "When?", and, if needed, the "How?" for the specific data point collected.

Figure 2.1 shows an example of a direct collection of the descriptive items for a given data point in a Case Report Form (CRF):

The "Who?" is Patient *0004* (sometimes referred to as "Subject") at clinical site *0021*. The "When?" is defaulted to *Visit 3* and specified more concretely to have occurred on July 21, 2024. The "What" suggests a *Systolic Blood Pressure* of *122 mmHG*, a *Diastolic Blood Pressure* of *86 mmHG*, and a *Pulse* of *68 beats/min*, and lastly the "How?" is defaulted to the *Supine Position*, but not further specifying which method or instrument was used for this blood pressure assessment.

So far so good . . . or not?

Even though blood pressure, as part of the overall routine vital signs assessments during clinical study visits, is a basic example, it serves well to illustrate the possible limitations to derive meaningful conclusions. Why do I say this?

Assuming that the site personnel conducting this blood pressure assessment actually followed all procedures correctly, such as ensuring the patient being in supine position, as well as using an acceptable and properly validated and calibrated blood pressure measurement device, there are still many possible gaps and questions.

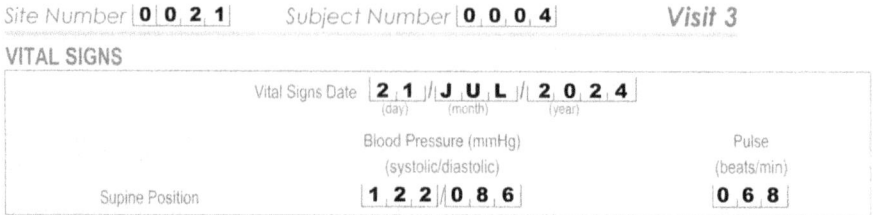

FIGURE 2.1
Example of CRF data collection.

How long was the patient in the supine position before measuring the blood pressure and which arm (right or left) was used?

The time of assessment is not being recorded, which in theory could suggest that the systolic blood pressure was 122 throughout the day, which would be nonsense.

Was the assessment done before or after taking the study medication?

The clinical protocol and CRF instructions might specify some of the assessment requirements; however, without any further evidence it will remain unknown if they have been followed.

Continuing this thought and the same example, let us assume that the true intent of the clinical protocol for this blood pressure assessment was to collect it:

- After the patient being 5 minutes in supine position and from the left arm
- Performed 30 minutes after intake of study medication
- At least 60 minutes after the last meal
- Using one of three permissible blood pressure measurement instruments

Not being able to reliably confirm for all blood pressure measurements and for all patients in this study that the clinical protocol requirements were followed 100% of the time means that the *122 mmHG systolic blood pressure* for patient *0004* at site *0021* on July 21, 2024, is nothing more than an attempt of an approximation to what the real value might have been.

Bearing in mind that systolic blood pressures can easily vary ±15% between arms, hours of day, body position during measurement, instruments used, and so on, and that we haven't even taken into account the possibility for human errors throughout the process, it is very likely that *122 mmHG* is not the true value we were looking for.

You might say, "Well, this is only a systolic blood pressure data point and with the volume of data across all patients and clinical sites, these errors might even out". This might be true; however, it is counting on the hope that the sum of all data errors does not skew results in any significant way.

Furthermore, let us not forget that this was just an example of systolic blood pressure. Every one of the thousands of data points for one subject and the millions of data points within a clinical study face the same dilemma and raise the same question – Does the recorded value actually represent the occurred reality?

It gets even more challenging with more subjective or historic data, such as the collection of AEs. If not reported immediately by the patient and only documented days or even weeks later at the actual study visit, important details around the event could go completely missing or captured incorrectly.

In the introduction of this chapter, I mentioned the development of the CDM mindset. Part of this development is the realization that the picture being created by the collected data for a given assessment, the patient, and the clinical study itself is only an approximation to real events that took place. It is our responsibility in CDM to make the gap between reality and the collected data that tries to describe this reality as small as possible. We will look at examples of how to use risk-based approaches and data analytics tools to accomplish this goal in the next chapters.

Some of you might already sense that the longer the time between the "occurrence of the recordable event or assessment" and the more steps required in the process to retrieve and capture the corresponding data, the bigger the gap will be between the ultimate truth and the collected data.

Derived from this realization the inherent value of ePROs, directly recorded data from sensors, or other forms of eSource data, becomes obvious. Even though deployment of these systems will also fall short from a 100% accurate representation of the ultimate truth, they do increase the probability of making the "truth gap" smaller. It will require thorough system validation, ample testing, and user training, before deployment, as well as continuous monitoring of incoming data to detect any systematic errors or anomalies.

One topic we have to address, even though it is an uncomfortable fact in our industry, is the area of actual fraud in clinical research. It can happen in all areas and by any party involved in the conduct of a clinical study. As this is a sensitive topic, I want to stay away from speculations and hypotheticals and rather share a real-life story of a personal experience related to identifying data fraud in a clinical study.

Example of Data Fraud in a Clinical Study

In January of 2007 I was part of a clinical team finalizing two Phase III studies intended for regulatory submission for a drug targeting hyperlipoproteinemia and vascular disease.

Shortly before database lock our company was alerted that the PI of one of our clinical sites in the study had received a warning letter from a regulatory agency.

As a proactive due diligent effort, our company decided to send a QA and a Clinical Operations representative together with me to Moscow, where the hospital was located.

Did I already mention that it was January?

Our assignment for the 6 days in Moscow was to review the clinical data originating from that site, interview all involved site personnel, and evaluate the local processes in terms of robustness.

After the first 4 days, we did not find any inconsistencies in the clinical data that rose to the level of creating suspicion, and the source data appeared to be complete and in line with the data recorded in the EDC system.

On the morning of Day 5, I did not expect it to become one of the most exciting days of my 30+-year career. Our team was starting to draft summary reports for our company, and we were wrapping up our personnel interviews. I wanted to use the time to have a look at the central laboratory

	A	B	C	D	E	F	G
1	scrnum	repno	accnum	labtst	tstresul	labunits	colldt
2	RU01-001	1	105018933	NET TRIGLYCERIDES	325	mg/dL	10/3/2005 00:00:00
3	RU01-001	2	105018933	TOTAL CHOLESTEROL	223	mg/dL	10/3/2005 00:00:00
4	RU01-001	3	105018933	HDL CHOLESTEROL	59	mg/dL	10/3/2005 00:00:00
5	RU01-001	4	105018933	TOTAL CHOL/HDL RATIO	3.8		10/3/2005 00:00:00
6	RU01-001	5	105018933	LDL/HDL CHOL RATIO	1.7		10/3/2005 00:00:00
7	RU01-001	6	105018933	NON-HDL CHOLESTEROL	164	mg/dL	10/3/2005 00:00:00
8	RU01-001	7	105018933	LDL CHOLESTEROL	99	mg/dL	10/3/2005 00:00:00
9	RU01-001	1	105019508	NET TRIGLYCERIDES	224	mg/dL	10/19/2005 00:00:00
10	RU01-001	2	105019508	TOTAL CHOLESTEROL	226	mg/dL	10/19/2005 00:00:00
11	RU01-001	3	105019508	HDL CHOLESTEROL	61	mg/dL	10/19/2005 00:00:00
12	RU01-001	4	105019508	TOTAL CHOL/HDL RATIO	3.7		10/19/2005 00:00:00
13	RU01-001	5	105019508	LDL/HDL CHOL RATIO	2.0		10/19/2005 00:00:00
14	RU01-001	6	105019508	NON-HDL CHOLESTEROL	165	mg/dL	10/19/2005 00:00:00
15	RU01-001	7	105019508	LDL CHOLESTEROL	120	mg/dL	10/19/2005 00:00:00
16	RU01-001	1	105016268	NET TRIGLYCERIDES	286	mg/dL	8/31/2005 00:00:00
17	RU01-001	2	105016268	TOTAL CHOLESTEROL	344	mg/dL	8/31/2005 00:00:00
18	RU01-001	3	105016268	HDL CHOLESTEROL	66	mg/dL	8/31/2005 00:00:00
19	RU01-001	4	105016268	TOTAL CHOL/HDL RATIO	5.2		8/31/2005 00:00:00
20	RU01-001	5	105016268	LDL/HDL CHOL RATIO	3.3		8/31/2005 00:00:00
21	RU01-001	6	105016268	NON-HDL CHOLESTEROL	278	mg/dL	8/31/2005 00:00:00
22	RU01-001	7	105016268	LDL CHOLESTEROL	221	mg/dL	8/31/2005 00:00:00
23	RU01-002	1	105018931	NET TRIGLYCERIDES	139	mg/dL	10/3/2005 00:00:00
24	RU01-002	2	105018931	TOTAL CHOLESTEROL	212	mg/dL	10/3/2005 00:00:00
25	RU01-002	3	105018931	HDL CHOLESTEROL	50	mg/dL	10/3/2005 00:00:00
26	RU01-002	4	105018931	TOTAL CHOL/HDL RATIO	4.2		10/3/2005 00:00:00
27	RU01-002	5	105018931	LDL/HDL CHOL RATIO	2.7		10/3/2005 00:00:00
28	RU01-002	6	105018931	NON-HDL CHOLESTEROL	162	mg/dL	10/3/2005 00:00:00
29	RU01-002	7	105018931	LDL CHOLESTEROL	134	mg/dL	10/3/2005 00:00:00
30	RU01-002	1	105019507	NET TRIGLYCERIDES	120	mg/dL	10/19/2005 00:00:00
31	RU01-002	2	105019507	TOTAL CHOLESTEROL	226	mg/dL	10/19/2005 00:00:00
32	RU01-002	3	105019507	HDL CHOLESTEROL	51	mg/dL	10/19/2005 00:00:00

FIGURE 2.2
Russian Central Laboratory Data Listing.

data, which I had left aside, because the primary focus had been on clinical data originating directly from that site.

I want to take you with me on the journey that I took through that laboratory data set, which I had loaded onto my laptop. These are the original screenshots I took while sitting in the hospital's review room that we had gotten assigned to.

First, I just scrolled through the laboratory data for all sites in Russia (this was 2007 so Excel was still state of the art, if you were wondering):

Nothing jumped out at me. At this stage I just wanted to get a "feeling" for the data and look for patterns, anything that looked different from a norm that I was still trying to define.

After a while I noticed that some of the collection dates for different subjects were identical, so I grouped clinical sites with a pivot table to show all the different collection dates by site and see how many patients had a laboratory sample taken on the same date.

This resulted in the following view. Site *RU02* was the one we were investigating:

Maybe not obvious immediately, but it seemed to me that the site we were investigating, *RU02*, had comparably more cases of multiple patients on the same day getting their blood sample taken for the central laboratory. There is nothing inherently suspicious about this fact, as it is not unusual for clinical research sites to treat multiple patients on the same day.

Nonetheless, it did prompt me to look closer at patients being treated on the same day. If you look at Figure 2.3 for site *RU02* and pick the sample collection date of January 23, 2006, you see that seven patients were at the site to give blood that day. Therefore, as a next step I created views in Excel putting pairs of patients and their respective laboratory values next to each other.

And this is when the goosebump moment happened. . . . Look at the following two original screenshots:

What you can clearly see in this first image is the pair of subjects *RU02–021 and RU02–25* side by side with their respective laboratory results.

And in the following image you can see the comparison of subjects RU02–030 and RU02–33.

I remember asking my Clinical Operations colleague how likely it was for two different people to have very similar laboratory data across dozens of

Count of tstresul	suir ▼							
colldt ▼	RU01	RU02	RU03	RU04	RU06	RU07	RU08	RU09
1/10/2006 00:00:00			2		1			
1/11/2006 00:00:00	4	2				2		
1/12/2006 00:00:00				2		2		1
1/13/2006 00:00:00		2						
1/16/2006 00:00:00	3	1						
1/17/2006 00:00:00	1		1			3		
1/18/2006 00:00:00		2						
1/19/2006 00:00:00				3			2	1
1/20/2006 00:00:00	3	3						
1/23/2006 00:00:00		7		1				
1/24/2006 00:00:00	5	1				1		
1/25/2006 00:00:00								2
1/26/2006 00:00:00	1	4	1	1	1			
1/27/2006 00:00:00		3						
1/3/2006 00:00:00								
1/30/2006 00:00:00						1	1	1
1/31/2006 00:00:00		3						
1/5/2006 00:00:00								
1/7/2006 00:00:00								
10/10/2005 00:00:00			2	2		1		
10/11/2005 00:00:00		1	1		1	2		4
10/12/2005 00:00:00					1	1	2	
10/13/2005 00:00:00	1	5	1	2	3		2	1
10/14/2005 00:00:00		9					4	
10/17/2005 00:00:00	6	2	2	2	2	3	1	
10/18/2005 00:00:00	2		2		2	3	1	3

FIGURE 2.3
Russian Central Laboratory Data Grouped by Sample Date.

	A	B	C	D	E	F	G		I	J	K	L	M	N
1	SCRNUM	ACCNUM	Coll-Date	LabTest	Result	Unit	Visit		SCRNUM	ACCNUM	Coll-Date	LabTest	Result	Unit
2	RU02-021	106001887	1/23/2006 00:	NET TRIGLYCERIDES	170	mg/dL	Week 4		RU02-025	106001889	1/23/2006 00:	NET TRIGLYCERIDES	167	mg/dL
3	RU02-021	106001887	1/23/2006 00:	TOTAL CHOLESTEROL	275	mg/dL	Week 4		RU02-025	106001889	1/23/2006 00:	TOTAL CHOLESTEROL	272	mg/dL
4	RU02-021	106001887	1/23/2006 00:	HDL CHOLESTEROL	66	mg/dL	Week 4		RU02-025	106001889	1/23/2006 00:	HDL CHOLESTEROL	66	mg/dL
5	RU02-021	106001887	1/23/2006 00:	TOTAL CHOL/HDL RATIO	4.2		Week 4		RU02-025	106001889	1/23/2006 00:	TOTAL CHOL/HDL RATIO	4.1	
6	RU02-021	106001887	1/23/2006 00:	LDL/HDL CHOL RATIO	2.7		Week 4		RU02-025	106001889	1/23/2006 00:	LDL/HDL CHOL RATIO	2.6	
7	RU02-021	106001887	1/23/2006 00:	NON-HDL CHOLESTEROL	209	mg/dL	Week 4		RU02-025	106001889	1/23/2006 00:	NON-HDL CHOLESTEROL	206	mg/dL
8	RU02-021	106001887	1/23/2006 00:	LDL CHOLESTEROL	175	mg/dL	Week 4		RU02-025	106001889	1/23/2006 00:	LDL CHOLESTEROL	173	mg/dL
9														
10	RU02-021	G562996	1/23/2006 00:	Basophils	0.18	GI/L	Week 4		RU02-025	G563025	1/23/2006 00:	Basophils	0.17	GI/L
11	RU02-021	G562996	1/23/2006 00:	Basophils (%)	1.4	%	Week 4		RU02-025	G563025	1/23/2006 00:	Basophils (%)	1.4	%
12	RU02-021	G562996	1/23/2006 00:	Eosinophils	0.26	GI/L	Week 4		RU02-025	G563025	1/23/2006 00:	Eosinophils	0.24	GI/L
13	RU02-021	G562996	1/23/2006 00:	Eosinophils (%)	2.0	%	Week 4		RU02-025	G563025	1/23/2006 00:	Eosinophils (%)	1.9	%
14	RU02-021	G562996	1/23/2006 00:	Hematocrit	0.47		Week 4		RU02-025	G563025	1/23/2006 00:	Hematocrit	0.48	
15	RU02-021	G562996	1/23/2006 00:	Hemoglobin	164	g/L	Week 4		RU02-025	G563025	1/23/2006 00:	Hemoglobin	165	g/L
16	RU02-021	G562996	1/23/2006 00:	Lymphocytes	3.27	GI/L	Week 4		RU02-025	G563025	1/23/2006 00:	Lymphocytes	3.11	GI/L
17	RU02-021	G562996	1/23/2006 00:	Lymphocytes (%)	25.5	%	Week 4		RU02-025	G563025	1/23/2006 00:	Lymphocytes (%)	25.1	%
18	RU02-021	G562996	1/23/2006 00:	MCH	35	pg	Week 4		RU02-025	G563025	1/23/2006 00:	MCH	34	pg
19	RU02-021	G562996	1/23/2006 00:	MCHC	350	g/L	Week 4		RU02-025	G563025	1/23/2006 00:	MCHC	344	g/L
20	RU02-021	G562996	1/23/2006 00:	MCV	99	fL	Week 4		RU02-025	G563025	1/23/2006 00:	MCV	99	fL
21	RU02-021	G562996	1/23/2006 00:	Monocytes	0.64	GI/L	Week 4		RU02-025	G563025	1/23/2006 00:	Monocytes	0.69	GI/L
22	RU02-021	G562996	1/23/2006 00:	Monocytes (%)	5.0	%	Week 4		RU02-025	G563025	1/23/2006 00:	Monocytes (%)	5.6	%
23	RU02-021	G562996	1/23/2006 00:	Neutrophils	8.45	GI/L	Week 4		RU02-025	G563025	1/23/2006 00:	Neutrophils	8.19	GI/L
24	RU02-021	G562996	1/23/2006 00:	Neutrophils (%)	66.0	%	Week 4		RU02-025	G563025	1/23/2006 00:	Neutrophils (%)	66.0	%
25	RU02-021	G562996	1/23/2006 00:	Platelets	307	GI/L	Week 4		RU02-025	G563025	1/23/2006 00:	Platelets	322	GI/L
26	RU02-021	G562996	1/23/2006 00:	RBC	4.7	TI/L	Week 4		RU02-025	G563025	1/23/2006 00:	RBC	4.9	TI/L
27	RU02-021	G562996	1/23/2006 00:	RBC Morphology	Normocytic		Week 4		RU02-025	G563025	1/23/2006 00:	RBC Morphology	Normocytic	
28	RU02-021	G562996	1/23/2006 00:	WBC	12.80	GI/L	Week 4		RU02-025	G563025	1/23/2006 00:	WBC	12.41	GI/L

	A	B	C	D	E	F	G		I	J	K	L	M	N
1	SCRNUM	ACCNUM	Coll-Date	LabTest	Result	Unit	Visit		SCRNUM	ACCNUM	Coll-Date	LabTest	Result	Unit
80	RU02-030	G563006	1/23/2006 00:	Phosphorus	3.4	mg/dL	Week 4		RU02-033	G563026	1/23/2006 00:	Phosphorus	3.3	mg/dL
81	RU02-030	G563006	1/23/2006 00:	Serum Uric Acid	7.5	mg/dL	Week 4		RU02-033	G563026	1/23/2006 00:	Serum Uric Acid	7.6	mg/dL
82	RU02-030	G563006	1/23/2006 00:	Urea Nitrogen	17	mg/dL	Week 4		RU02-033	G563026	1/23/2006 00:	Urea Nitrogen	18	mg/dL
83	RU02-030	G563006	1/23/2006 00:	Urea Nitrogen/Creat Ratio	16.9		Week 4		RU02-033	G563026	1/23/2006 00:	Urea Nitrogen/Creat Ratio	17.7	
84	RU02-030	G563006	1/23/2006 00:	AST (SGOT)	26	U/L	Week 4		RU02-033	G563026	1/23/2006 00:	AST (SGOT)	23	U/L
85	RU02-030	G563006	1/23/2006 00:	ALT (SGPT)	15	U/L	Week 4		RU02-033	G563026	1/23/2006 00:	ALT (SGPT)	13	U/L
86	RU02-030	G563006	1/23/2006 00:	Creatinine (Rate Blanked)	1.0	mg/dL	Week 4		RU02-033	G563026	1/23/2006 00:	Creatinine (Rate Blanked)	1.0	mg/dL
87	RU02-030	G563006	1/23/2006 00:	Direct Bilirubin	0.1	mg/dL	Week 4		RU02-033	G563026	1/23/2006 00:	Direct Bilirubin	0.2	mg/dL
88	RU02-030	G563006	1/23/2006 00:	Calcium (EDTA)	10.1	mg/dL	Week 4		RU02-033	G563026	1/23/2006 00:	Calcium (EDTA)	10.2	mg/dL
89	RU02-030	G563006	1/23/2006 00:	Serum Chloride	104	mEq/L	Week 4		RU02-033	G563026	1/23/2006 00:	Serum Chloride	103	mEq/L
90	RU02-030	G563006	1/23/2006 00:	Serum Bicarbonate	28.7	mEq/L	Week 4		RU02-033	G563026	1/23/2006 00:	Serum Bicarbonate	27.2	mEq/L
91	RU02-030	G563006	1/23/2006 00:	Serum Potassium	4.3	mEq/L	Week 4		RU02-033	G563026	1/23/2006 00:	Serum Potassium	4.4	mEq/L
92	RU02-030	G563006	1/23/2006 00:	Serum Sodium	143	mEq/L	Week 4		RU02-033	G563026	1/23/2006 00:	Serum Sodium	143	mEq/L
93	RU02-030	G563006	1/23/2006 00:	LDH	210	U/L	Week 4		RU02-033	G563026	1/23/2006 00:	LDH	192	U/L
94	RU02-030	G563006	1/23/2006 00:	Alkaline Phosphatase	95	U/L	Week 4		RU02-033	G563026	1/23/2006 00:	Alkaline Phosphatase	95	U/L
95	RU02-030	G563006	1/23/2006 00:	Creatine Kinase	136	U/L	Week 4		RU02-033	G563026	1/23/2006 00:	Creatine Kinase	118	U/L
96	RU02-030	G563006	1/23/2006 00:	Albumin	4.4	g/dL	Week 4		RU02-033	G563026	1/23/2006 00:	Albumin	4.4	g/dL
97	RU02-030	G563006	1/23/2006 00:	Total Protein	7.8	g/dL	Week 4		RU02-033	G563026	1/23/2006 00:	Total Protein	7.8	g/dL
98	RU02-030	G563006	1/23/2006 00:	Serum Glucose	115	mg/dL	Week 4		RU02-033	G563026	1/23/2006 00:	Serum Glucose	119	mg/dL
99	RU02-030	G563006	1/23/2006 00:	Total Bilirubin	0.7	mg/dL	Week 4		RU02-033	G563026	1/23/2006 00:	Total Bilirubin	0.7	mg/dL
100	RU02-030	G563006	1/23/2006 00:	Serum Amylase	59	U/L	Week 4		RU02-033	G563026	1/23/2006 00:	Serum Amylase	59	U/L

FIGURE 2.4

Russian Central Laboratory Data – Fraud identified! Looking closely, you will see that the respective values for the same laboratory parameters are very similar.

parameters. She responded that it was extremely unlikely for this to be the case. At that point in time, I had already identified 26 (!) matching pairs at site *RU02* and zero at any other site. Case closed beyond any reasonable doubt.

But the question remained. What did the site and the PI actually do to result in these matching pairs of laboratory data?

When we confronted the PI with the evidence, after initial denying, she did confess and explained that many visits at site *RU02* were rushed with the goal of getting as many patients as possible. During blood samples, the site coordinators conducting the blood samples were trying to save time by taking blood only from one patient but then putting it in multiple tubes and labeling those with other patient's IDs, which explained why tubes with blood seemingly originating from different patients would have almost identical results. The small variances in the final data can be attributed to the laboratory margins of error.

There is so much to unpack and learn from this example.

First and foremost, we see here a case where source data turned out to be incorrect due to fraud committed by site personnel, showing that even the most desirable form of clinical data, that is, source, cannot be trusted blindly.

The question can also be raised whether this particular data integrity issue could or should have been identified sooner. If you recall the dates from the screenshots, most laboratory samples from site *RU02* were taken in January of 2006. That data was in the clinical database shortly thereafter. We only found the issue a year later at the clinical site. Did the IDRP fail?

We have to remember that in 2006 sophisticated data analytics tools were not in existence yet, and more advanced review in the form of "lack of variability between patient data" was barely used.

Wrapping up this data fraud example, it also shows the ever-evolving knowledge base for CDM, which allows us to learn from these incidences and improve our IDRPs and data analytics tools and programming approaches to incorporate new reviews that will identify data patterns as the one seen in this example.

The PI from site RU02 was criminally charged and will never be able to conduct clinical studies again. All the data from this site was left in the overall dataset, but excluded from the analysis, as we could not rule out broader misconduct for other data domains at this site.

Lastly, let us not forget that the inability to achieve 100% accuracy for a clinical study is understood and accepted by all regulatory agencies. The aim is to achieve an aggregated final clinical data set that can support the predefined analysis. From a less idealistic and more pragmatic CDM perspective, the focus should be on avoidance of systematic errors, continuous risk assessments of incoming data, and trend analysis to detect signals in the data that might require corrective actions.

Atoms in the Universe

In the previous paragraphs we looked into some of the inherent complexities around collecting clinical data that is hopefully painting an adequate picture of real events.

We are now taking an even more daring plunge into the almost infinite volume of clinical data. I want to forewarn you that throughout this section there might arise the occasional sentiment of resignation in the face of the seemingly impossible task to deal with the immensity of the clinical data volume and variety we have to confront. Rest assured that I will not leave you without concrete approaches and solutions on how to deal with this task and identify the actual areas to focus on to eliminate the background noise.

The number of clinical data points being collected in a given study varies by phase, overall size, and therapeutic area. Suggested ranges for this number that I have seen start in the thousands for very small Phase I studies, up to several million data points for massive Phase III studies with thousands of patients.

Let us do our own calculation taking an average 200 patient study with 10 scheduled visits and a CRF with 20 forms per visit with 25 data points per form. If all patients were to complete all forms and all visits, we would collect 200 patients × 10 visits × 20 forms × 25 data points, resulting in a total of one million data points. As clinical data originating from CRFs accounts for less than 50% of the total data in clinical studies, it is a conservative estimate that in our hypothetical study another million data points will be collected from non-CRF data, which is often referred to as "external data". These are your central and specialty laboratory data sets, patient questionnaires, adjudication data for images or other endpoint related assessments, and so on. Bringing our total number of data points for this average study to 2 million. Two million!

How do you deal from a CDM point of view with 2 million data points and the mandate to ensure that they will get collected and reviewed adequately to reflect reality?

Let us start by trying to visualize how 2 million data points look like.

As part of a session on AI and ML I chaired at the 2024 SCDM EMEA Forum (www.scdm.org), I was providing a similar introduction to the topic and used the following image to put 2 million dots, each one of them representing one clinical data point, on the screen.

Each square contains 100 × 100 dots for a total of 10,000 dots per square. The entire image contains 10 × 20 squares, bringing the total number of dots to 2 million.

We can now link this image to our sample study and run through examples on how visual representations of clinical data would manifest themselves. As a reminder, the goal of this approach is to look at CDMs' remit through different lenses, learn about different perspectives into clinical data, and get a true feeling for the volume of it.

We are now overlaying a clinical site structure, representing the participating research hospitals, for our sample study, to the image. Each of the 50 small squares in Figure 2.6 shall represent one of the participating clinical sites. In the real world, patients and corresponding data points would not be perfectly distributed like this, but for illustration purposes and the arguments to be made, this suffices.

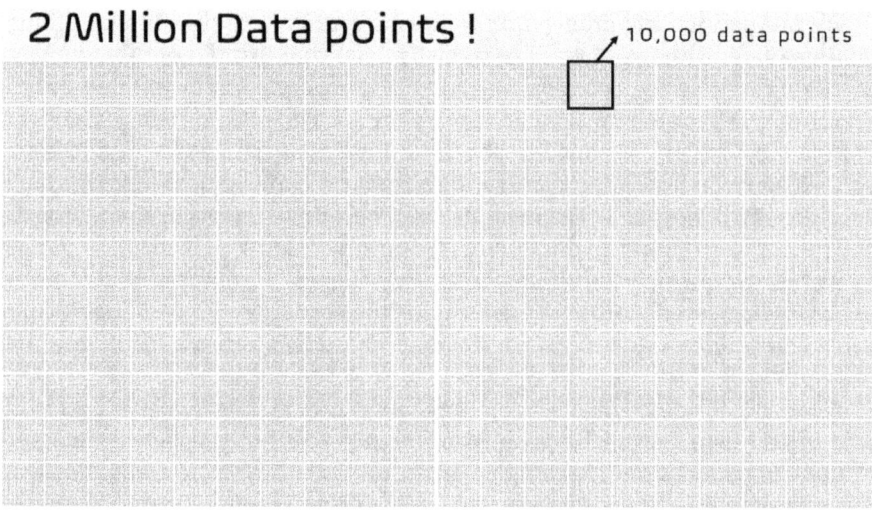

FIGURE 2.5
Two million data points.

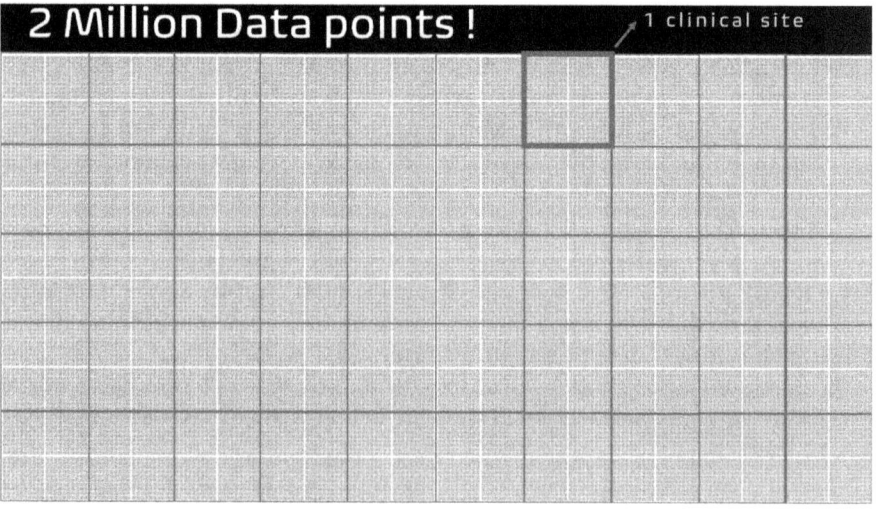

FIGURE 2.6
Two million data points distributed between 50 clinical sites.

This is obviously just the framework. Now it will get really interesting when we fill this visual representation of clinical data with some meaning.

Let us start with Figure 2.7 showing all of the AE data as it may have occurred in this study, by highlighting all the AE-related data points, for example, AE verbatim term, AE start date, intensity and their distribution within each site.

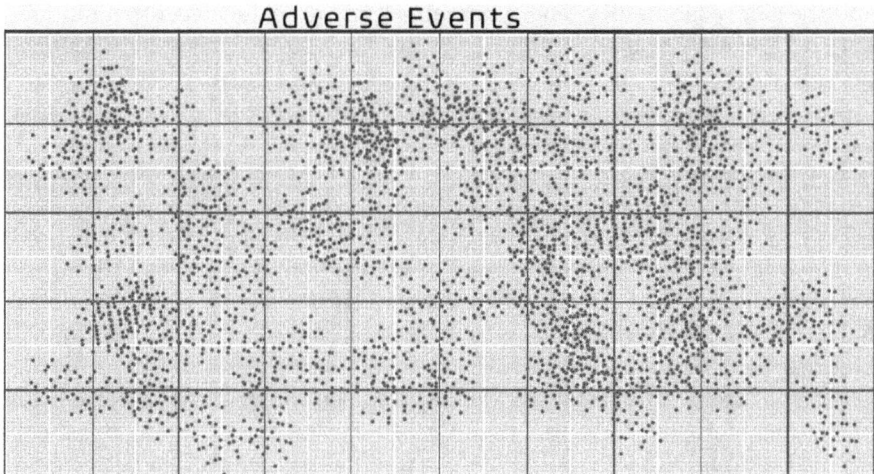

FIGURE 2.7
Illustration of AE data distribution.

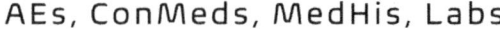

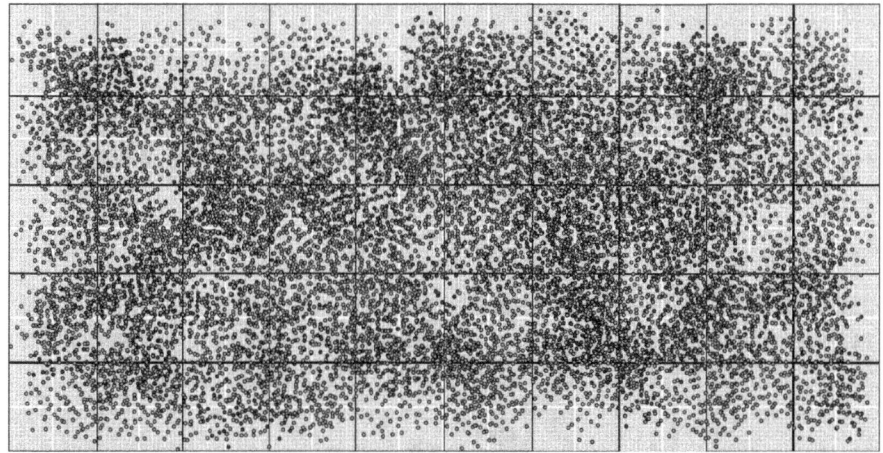

FIGURE 2.8
Illustration of AE, ConMed, MedHis, and Safety Lab data distribution.

Even though this is only an illustration, we can identify very quickly clinical sites with more AEs than other sites. The location within a square could indicate different onset times or other possible patterns. We will get back to the topic of patterns very shortly. First, however, let us get to the final visualization of how multiple data domains may be related, and part of the standard aggregated reviews would show up in an image like this.

In Figure 2.8, you can see the combination of AE data together with the data domains of concomitant medication (ConMeds), medical history (MedHis), and the safety laboratory. These domains undergo extensive, often manual, data review efforts to ensure, for example, that every concomitant medication has a corresponding match in the AE or medical history data set.

Yes, it looks and is very chaotic. Just going by Figure 2.7 or 2.8, no correlations or trends seem to be identifiable.

Let me get you in on a little secret. When I was creating these images, I started with a few random dots, which I grouped together exactly as in Figure 2.9. I then just copied the same group of dots and rotated, mirrored, and overlayed them multiple times to create the seemingly random and chaotic images you saw before. However, all the seemingly chaotic distribution from the previous images was created by one sole pattern – the one in Figure 2.9.

As it is almost impossible to identify and see the original pattern in the preceding overlayed pictures, I used the same original distribution from earlier and highlighted four of the many examples of the original pattern hidden in the sea of data points in Figure 2.10.

So, what is the point of this exercise? Even though these are only hypothetical scenarios, it is easy to imagine that repeating data patterns like this can occur in any clinical study. The specific pattern in this example could represent an AE, like "Migraine", which occurs within a certain time window

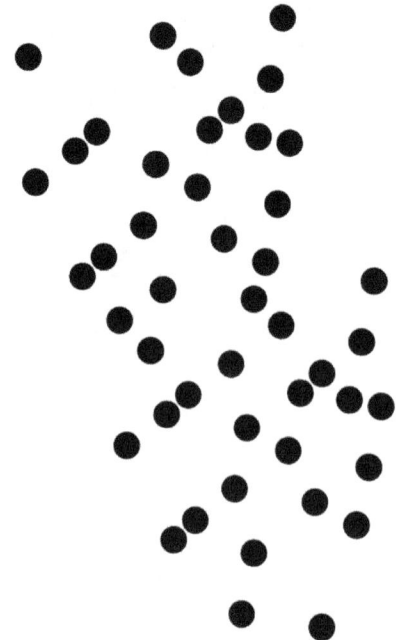

FIGURE 2.9
Random dots representing clinical data.

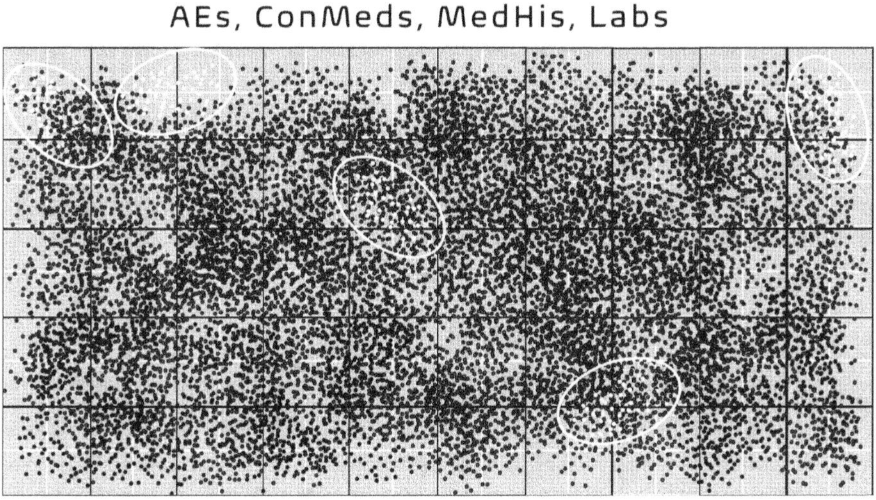

AEs, ConMeds, MedHis, Labs

FIGURE 2.10
Showing examples of the original pattern hidden in the data chaos (darker dots in the white ovals).

after study-medication dosing, but only in patients with a specific medical history. These correlations could remain hidden, if data is only looked at on the item or single patient level.

Yes, clinical data review typically also groups data by domains to categorize AEs by frequency, possible relationship to study medications, or other standard reconciliation activities; however, the possible number of correlations is so unimaginably huge, which should leave us all wondering about "What are we possibly missing?"

This brings us to one of the main items and considerations for this chapter.

We already got a sense from the images in the previous paragraphs that we are dealing with a huge volume of possible data correlations and subsets. But how big is this number and what does it mean for us from a practical point of view?

The first part of the question has a relatively straightforward mathematical answer. If we continue with the previously established assumption of 2 million clinical data points in an average clinical study, the number of possible subsets of a (data)set of 2 million items equals $2^{2,000,000} - 1$, which is an unimaginably large number.

Nevertheless, just for fun, let us try to compare this number to something more "tangible". According to universetoday.com the number of atoms in the known universe is estimated to be somewhere between 10^{78} and 10^{82}. For argument's sake let us pick the middle of the range and go with 10^{80} atoms. A few galaxies more or less won't make a difference.

Applying some basic math, we transform $2^{2,000,000}$ to a base "10" number:

Solving for X: $10^X = 2^{2,000,000}$

Apply $\log_{10}$ on both sides: $\log_{10}(10^X) = \log_{10}(2^{2,000,000})$

Apply log-rules $\log_a(a^b) = b$, and $\log_a(b^c) = c \cdot \log_a(b)$, giving us: $X = 2,000,000 \cdot \log_{10}(2)$

Calculate $\log_{10}(2)$: $X = 2,000,000 \cdot 0.301029995\ldots$

Giving us the final result: $X \approx 602060$

Therefore, $2^{2,000,000}$ is approximately 10^{602060}, which is a "1" followed by 602060 "0"s compared to the number of atoms in our universe which is *only* a "1" followed by about 80 "0"s.

I remember the first time I saw the order of magnitude difference between these two numbers and feeling overwhelmed by the abyss of the infinite possible unknown patterns that might exist in the clinical data of a given study.

One more number play, before we look at what possible practical ramifications this might have for CDM and our industry.

Some people will rightly point out that the vast majority of the possible 10^{602060} subsets in our clinical study are nonsensical and will not reveal any valuable medical information or contribute to identifying and risk areas. This is undoubtedly correct as there will be subsets containing, for example, one patient's age together with some of the laboratory results from another patient, paired with the intensity of an unrelated AE. Nothing meaningful can be derived from these sorts of subsets. However, and this is the point I like to argue with my statistical friends and colleagues, we have to look at the immense size of the overall number of possibilities. Even if 99.9999 . . . (insert here 601970 more "9"s) . . . 9999% of all the subsets were nonsense, we are still left with about 10^{80} subsets (wait, this number sounds familiar – right the atoms in the universe!) that could possibly contain meaningful new insights for us.

In the end, it does not matter if the number of subsets containing patterns that can reveal meaningful insights for us is 10^{80} or 10^{10} or 10 or just 1. We just don't know what is hiding in this infinite sea of clinical data links and we have to ask ourselves – Can we afford not knowing? Are we putting patients at risks and can these risks be identified earlier and prevented? Or are we missing hidden benefits of investigational drugs that could improve patient's lives today?

One thing, though, that we do know for sure, by looking at clinical data from this angle and having in mind how much of clinical data review is still being done manually through listing reviews or item-by-item SDV by CRAs, is that we are not even scratching the surface of the information treasure we have in front of us.

We cannot reach the stars by building a ladder. We need a novel approach, a paradigm-shift in our thinking that puts clinical data in the focus of R&D spending, and we have to start unleashing the full power of the ML/AI-driven technology environment that we have finally at our fingertips.

The Power of the Audit Trail

The audit trail is an essential part of every clinical system that collects and processes clinical data.

Within the 21CFR Part 11 regulatory framework the FDA clearly states that "it may nonetheless be important to have audit trails or other physical, logical, or procedural security measures in place to ensure the trustworthiness and reliability of the records" and that "Audit trails can be particularly appropriate when users are expected to create, modify, or delete regulated records during normal operation" (FDA Part 11, Electronic Records – Guidance for Industry, Paragraph III, Part B, Section 2, https://www.fda.gov/regulatory-information/search-fda-guidance-documents/part-11-electronic-records-electronic-signatures-scope-and-application).

Representatives from regulatory agencies around the globe have increased their efforts in the last years to include audit trail review (ATR) as part of their routine inspection agendas. They must have realized the power of the information collected and accumulating in the audit trails throughout the conduct of a clinical study.

Let us look at the fundamental components of audit trails using EDC as an example. At its core, the audit trail can be seen as a logbook documenting any activity in the EDC system. Depending on which EDC system you are using there might be different approaches to how to structure the audit trail data.

The two main parts are:

- Any activity that creates, changes, or deletes a clinical data record
- Any activity by users or the system itself executing available functionality

The first part includes documenting the original manual entry or automated load of a new clinical record, covering the What? Who? When? How? thus providing the clinical data information that was entered or loaded, the UserID identifying the person who did it, a time stamp documenting when the action took place, and lastly the method of entry.

Any subsequent change to this data point will not only create a new record in the audit trail capturing the same information as the original record but also store the previous and new value. Records in the audit trail can be quite lengthy as they also contain many more references to the metadata being in play for a given new entry or change to existing data. The essence of the information though is the aforementioned group of What? Who? When? How? which enable reviewers to reconstruct the trajectory of all clinical data in this specific system.

The second part of the audit trail captures the activities of the different users and roles to which they are assigned. Typical activities captured are:

- Creation of queries originating from the execution of the IDRP
- Logging in and out of the system
- Changing database statuses through flags such as "Freeze", "Lock", and "Source Data Verified (SDV)"
- Running of reports
- Exporting data
- Any other activity permissible in the system, which does not add new data or change existing data, as that would be captured as described in the first part of the audit trail

Now that we have established the basic content and functionality of the audit trail, we can look into the surely more interesting aspect of why regulatory auditors are so keen to review it and what valuable information can be derived for CDM and other functions to support risk-based quality management.

Starting with some examples from the regulatory inspector point of view. These examples can be very helpful as knowing them can put CDM departments in the position to address these items a priori rather than being faced with them after the fact during an audit.

To enable you to start the discussion around ATR at your company we will look at the following list of examples:

- Time stamps
- Log-in frequency and time
- Number of data changes for a given data point
- Data changes after SDV

Time Stamps

Looking at specific data domains, such as patient report data and the corresponding time stamps documenting when those records were created, puts the reviewer in a position to check for suspicious patterns and adherence to protocol requirements. As an example, if a patient questionnaire is required to be completed after dinner and before bedtime, the time stamp for this record will show how closely patients followed the instructions.

A related example I have seen being flagged by auditors is the recording of certain clinical assessments, which by definition have a minimum duration, for example, a 5-minute treadmill walk for which start and end time are being recorded. If patterns emerge for certain patients or clinical sites that suggest requirements specified in the protocol were not adhered to, it will raise flags to possibly investigate further to see data integrity has been compromised.

Log-in Frequency and Time

PIs, or their documented designees, are accountable for reviewing the data for their respective clinical sites, before they endorse the entire content with an electronic signature. Even though this review should happen throughout the conduct of the clinical study, it has become almost the norm for PIs to log in at the end of the study to perform the electronic signature task and log off within minutes, opening the door for the question of how is it possible for this PI to review and endorse all patient data within that time.

Both examples above can, and probably should, be part of a standardized ATR process in every CDM department.

Number of Data Changes for a Given Data Point

The ideal scenario for clinical data is to originate from a correctly conducted clinical assessment and captured unaltered and correctly in the electronic system of choice with no need to ever change again.

Unfortunately, not all data points follow this journey. Through the process of data review by CDM and all the other roles performing the same task, as described in the previous chapter, 1000s of queries are being issued and directed at clinical sites or laboratories to doublecheck or question the validity of some of these datapoints.

Within reason, meaning based on a pre-defined IDRP, such review activities are necessary and will identify erroneous data that then can be corrected. Seeing clinical data changes in the audit trail is perfectly fine, if, and only if, these changes go hand in hand with a documented reason for the change. However, it does and should raise suspicion, if the same data point changes its value multiple times. Especially if the data point in question is related to the primary or secondary endpoints evaluated in the study.

Underlying causes for data points changing multiple times can be overlapping data review activities with the result of contradicting queries being issued and confusing clinical site personnel. Another reason could be query-texts that are worded in a leading way biasing site personnel toward different answers. Any of these reasons are bad and should be avoided at all costs.

Therefore, I recommend having a "data change counter" on every clinical data point and an audit trail report that flags any items that have been changed twice or more. This report should be grouped by clinical site and data domain to easily identify patterns and concrete actions to follow up to identify the issue at hand.

Data Changes After SDV

Keeping my favorite one for last. The topic of SDV is controversial in our industry, and we will go into more detail on it in later chapters. For the purpose of this discussion around audit trails, let us focus on the fact that clinical studies will have a clinical monitoring plan in place, created by Clinical Operations, defining the level of SDV planned for the study at hand.

This plan will specify which patients, data domains, and clinical data points will need to be SDVed, as we say, by the CRAs. It could be all data points or just a percentage thereof.

As a reminder, performing SDV is the challenging task of performing SDR and then ensuring that the *source data* has been captured correctly in EDC. When the CRA has reviewed the source and confirmed that the entry in EDC mirrors the information in the source, they confirm and document their review by applying an SDV flag to the corresponding data points in EDC.

So far so good, and coming to the key question now:

How is it possible that clinical data changes occur in EDC *after* SDV has been performed by the CRA?

This should never happen! If the source data is the ultimate documented truth of the clinical assessment and the CRA confirmed with the flag that the data in EDC is identical, no query, no reviewer, and no change of plans should be able to trigger a data change, as according to the CRA the truth has been documented.

Similar to my suggestion of a standard report for items with two or more data changes, I even more emphatically suggest implementing a report flagging all data changes that occurred after SDV.

The only logical explanations, which are not "pretty", for such a scenario are:

- The CRAs made a mistake or just clicked the SDV flag without performing SDV
- Systematic issues around the documented source data at time of creation
- Biased clinical data review resulting in sites changing data because of subjective and leading query texts
- Incomplete source data at time of CRA review, raising the question of clinical site's ability to create reliable, complete, and contemporaneous source data

CRAs are humans and mistakes happen. Time spent at clinical sites by CRAs is precious, and the pressure on CRAs is immense to do myriads of things. I am pointing this out, as I do not want to paint the CRAs as the culprits. Insufficient resources and conflicting priorities can result in more human errors. Therefore, I do see the audit trail report showing "Data changes after SDV" as a help for Clinical Operations to identify the problem areas for CRAs, sites, and possible systematic issues.

These are four specific examples (Time Stamp, Log-in frequency and time, Number of data changes for a given data point, and Data changes after SDV), which provide extremely valuable insights by using data from the audit trail.

It has not yet become standard practice for many CDM departments to incorporate this kind of data review in their standard processes; however, inspectors from regulatory agencies have added the audit trail onto their list of items to check more routinely during audits.

Therefore, I do recommend CDM departments to expand their respective IDRPs to include a reference to standardized analytical reviews of the audit trail. In addition to the four examples shared earlier, the following list is a good starting point for amplifying ATR and as a result increase overall robustness of clinical data and regulatory inspection readiness:

- Number of distinct user IDs (to check user access management)
- Entry date/time compared to assessment date/time (to rank sites by entry cycle time)
- Reasons provided for changing data (system or user generated? Are reasons plausible?)
- Timing and scope of structural changes to the database (including risk of data loss/unexpected changes due to these changes)

This list can be expanded as new risk areas are being identified for your company or for a concrete study. If you implement the ATR mechanisms for the total of eight examples provided in this section, you will have a very solid foundation for identifying possible risks early on, by using the audit trail.

And, when sitting in front of the regulatory inspector during an audit and being asked about your approach to ATR, you will have at least something to show and say, compared to the current prominent answer of "Oops!"

The Case for AI in CDM

Throughout this chapter we have seen examples of data fraud, unimaginable volumes of data, and the complexity of performing clinical data review in a clinical study. These examples raise the question whether there is even a need to make a case for AI in CDM, as it should already be obvious that traditional approaches are falling short in front of the challenges of modern clinical studies.

Looking at the seven Vs of big data, that is, Volume, Velocity, Variety, Variability, Veracity, Value, and Visualization, we see that especially the first three Vs (Volume, Velocity, and Variety) have grown to such levels of complexity that humans equipped with just listings, static edit checks, and a few visualizations are exposed to missing crucial risk indicators, or unexpected benefit signals in a clinical study.

On the flip side, deploying head over heels an AI-labeled review machinery in the hope for miracle outcomes without adequate human expert oversight will likely have even more disastrous consequences.

So what do we do?

We can start by trusting the solid foundation that has been built over the last decades, including the more supportive regulatory framework, as well as existing technologies and processes that have earned the label "best practice". It is and will continue to be important for CDM professionals to maintain a healthy portion of skepticism, now when every industry sector and technology solution comes with the label "Powered by AI".

In Figure 2.11, we do not need AI to tell us to look at the *Heart Rate* for this patient at *Visit 5*, because our traditional methods already identify these out-of-range values easily as part of the standard data review practices. The detection of this outlier is not AI!

However, I wonder if you noticed the actual odd observation in the chart that our traditional review would not pick up, but a trained AI tool could possibly flag?

Do you see it?

It seems odd that all 10 observations are even numbers which are divisible by 3, or in other words – all numbers are multiples of 6. Considering that only every 6th number has this characteristic, there is a chance of only 1/6 or ≈16.7% for this to be the case for a random number.

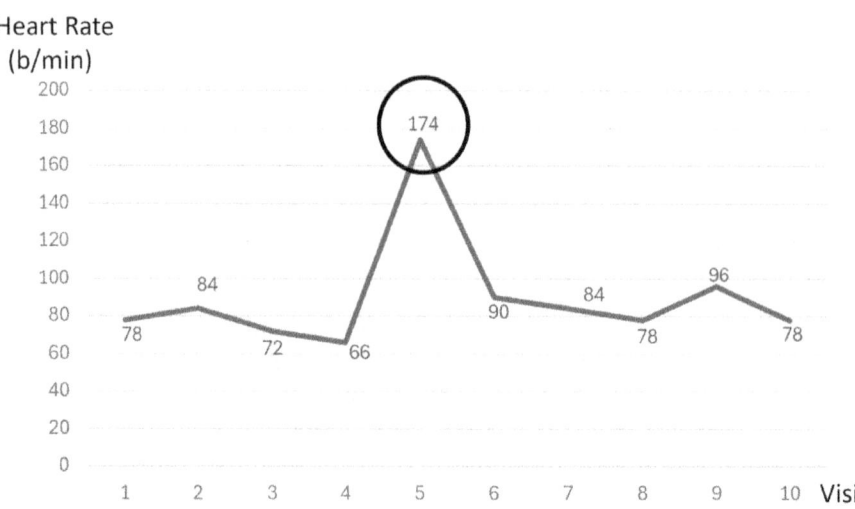

FIGURE 2.11
Hypothetical Heart Rate Graph.

Heart rate cannot be considered a purely random number as the values are bound within a certain range, which is compatible with life and follows a bell curve distribution within that range. However, within that bell curve there should be no preference for a certain number type. Thus, the random chance of 10 consecutive heart rate values over the span of 10 visits to be all multiples of 6 is $(1/6)^{10}$ or 0.00000165381%. Looks unlikely to me to happen by chance and worth investigating in terms of comparison to other patients and considering an inspection of the device measuring the heart rate at that site.

This was just one example of many possible mathematical considerations for deployment of AI-based review to see if the clinical data we are looking at is:

- Random or not random enough
- Possibly too perfect (suggesting system errors or fabricated data)
- Being rounded up or down by a system

To address the current hype around AI, we should differentiate between truly amazing insights we can only gain through the deployment of AI and those that just drive efficiency, but don't provide new knowledge we can use to advance science.

Let me use a basic analogy. Using a car to get from *A* to *B* is without any doubt more time-efficient than walking; however, as a human I would have reached the same destination eventually as well, just needing more time for it. Therefore, we have not considered cars to be artificially intelligent, but still very useful.

However, while driving from *A* to *B* with an AI-equipped car, I am about to get involved in an accident and the car proactively reads the situation, takes over control, and avoids the accident, and the situation changes. Something happened here because of my limited human senses, inability to recognize the pattern of danger early enough, reaction time, data processing capabilities, lack of computing power to evaluate all possible options, and so on. I, as human, was not up to the task to avoid this accident. AI, however, used its trained algorithms to perform a superhuman task.

This brings us back to the overall mission for CDM and the daily tasks at hand. The promise of AI, as I see it, is to unleash it on the unknown-to-human patterns in our clinical databases. Not just for the one clinical study we are working on, but for the entirety of clinical programs and accumulated knowledge from decades of clinical research.

The earthshattering impact this can have on our entire industry and healthcare systems globally is immense. Clinical trials could run much faster as the target patient groups would already be identified and clinical data would reveal new, never before considered or imagined, information.

Moving from paper to EDC was a significant step, and adjustment, for our industry in the late 1990s and early 2000s, followed by widespread use of ePRO systems and decentralization efforts. The promise of AI, however, if we get it right as an industry, and possibly humankind, will be a bigger quantum leap for us, than all of the previous advancements together.

Summary

What a journey! We looked at clinical data from some new perspectives and saw that some of the information in front of us cannot always be taken at face value.

The main goal of this chapter was to "train" our CDM mindset, by looking at the full range of data from the single data point of 122 mmHG systolic blood pressure, to getting lost in the abyss of uncountable subsets of data and their hidden messages, lurking behind unrecognizable for human patterns, for which we will have to deploy sophisticated AI technologies to be able to see and understand.

We also saw examples of how to follow one's gut feeling when with our currently available analytical tools we identify data oddities, which could just happen by chance or be the early warning sign of a bigger risk.

Lastly, we looked at the often-neglected audit trail and its importance for ensuring data integrity beyond the clinical data sets and to be prepared for regulatory audits in this regard, and we started to tip our toe into the AI discussion, which will accompany us through a few more chapters down the road.

We will now have to put our new insights to use, when we continue to the next stage of our CDM journey – Risk-Based Quality Management (RBQM) and why CDM should lead it.

3

Demystifying Risk-Based Quality Management (RBQM) and Why CDM Should Lead It

With Joanna Florek-Marwitz and Osnat Mamet

We are now moving on to one of the key areas related to ensuring regulatory compliance and quality delivery for clinical trials – RBQM.

With the knowledge gained from the two previous chapters around positioning CDM, getting a deeper understanding of the complexities around clinical data, and starting to develop the CDM mindset, we are now ready to put this knowledge to practical use.

In this chapter we will reference the regulatory guidance framework as it relates to RBQM, and how to put the building stones of RBQM, such as Quality by Design (QbD), Critical to Success Factors, and QTLs in place.

Part of the "demystification" will also address the still existing confusion in daily dialogues between RBQM and Risk-Based Monitoring (RBM).

This will be another exciting journey with concrete examples and key take home messages for you to use in your effort to either start building or further expanding and improving your RBQM leadership role at your respective company.

Concretely we will cover:

- Cornerstones of RBQM
- Risk-Based Quality Management – What risks? Who manages?
- The case for CDM's Lead role in RBQM

Cornerstones of RBQM

Let's Start with QA – So We Don't Forget It

In the intricate landscape of clinical trials, where every data point holds the potential to shape patient safety and trial success, RBQM emerges as a beacon of proactive assurance. RBQM transcends the traditional reactive approaches to QA by focusing on identifying, assessing, and mitigating risks throughout the trial lifecycle.

However, the implementation of RBQM cannot be fully realized without the integral involvement of QA teams. It is imperative to recognize and embed QA as a foundational element in the RBQM process.

At the heart of RBQM lies a comprehensive understanding of the regulatory landscape governing clinical trials. Regulatory authorities such as the U.S. Food and Drug Administration (FDA) and the European Medicines Agency (EMA) mandate stringent guidelines to ensure data integrity, patient safety, and regulatory compliance. These guidelines, including ICH E6(R2) and (R3) and ICH E8 (R1), emphasize the importance of risk-based approaches to quality management, underscoring the need for systematic risk identification and mitigation strategies. QA teams bring an in-depth knowledge of these regulations and ensure that all RBQM activities align with these standards, thus safeguarding the trial against regulatory breaches.

QA professionals are trained to anticipate potential risks before they materialize, leveraging their expertise to foresee and address issues that could compromise data quality or patient safety. Their involvement ensures that risk assessments are thorough and that mitigation strategies are robust, reducing the likelihood of trial disruptions and enhancing the overall reliability of trial outcomes.

It is crucial to emphasize that this knowledge and way of thinking should not be exclusive to QA. The QA mindset should be adopted by many stakeholders within the organization, especially those involved in RBQM. Sharing day-to-day work with QA can leverage and strengthen the rationale behind their work.

The meticulous nature of QA processes ensures that all data collected is accurate, consistent, and complete. By embedding QA into the RBQM process, clinical trials can achieve higher standards of data integrity, which is crucial for making informed decisions about drug safety and efficacy. This level of scrutiny helps in maintaining the credibility of the trial data, which is paramount for regulatory submissions and subsequent market approval.

QA's role extends beyond compliance; it fosters a culture of continuous improvement within the organization. By consistently monitoring and evaluating processes, QA teams can identify areas for enhancement and drive process optimization initiatives. This proactive stance not only improves current trial outcomes but also sets a higher benchmark for future studies, promoting a sustainable quality-focused mindset across the organization.

The integration of QA in the RBQM framework promotes stronger cross-functional collaboration between different departments, including clinical operations, data management, and regulatory affairs. QA acts as a bridge, ensuring that all stakeholders are aligned on quality objectives. This collaborative approach enhances the efficiency and effectiveness of the trial process, leading to better outcomes and a more cohesive work environment.

In conclusion, the RBQM process is incomplete without QA involvement. It is not merely beneficial but essential for ensuring regulatory compliance, enhancing data integrity, promoting continuous improvement, and fostering a culture of collaboration and proactive risk management. Recognizing and elevating the role of QA within the clinical trials industry is crucial for driving the cultural change needed to achieve higher standards of quality and reliability in clinical studies. The success of the process relies on the engagement of many stakeholders, but the mindset must be ingrained within the organization from a QA perspective, addressing challenges through a comprehensive view of total risk management.

Critical to Quality

In the realm of RBQM, the concept of Critical to Quality (CTQ) plays a pivotal role in ensuring the attainment of trial objectives and endpoints with utmost precision and reliability. CTQs encompass critical processes and data elements that directly influence the quality, efficacy, and safety of clinical trial outcomes, particularly in the context of a study's primary objectives and endpoints.

These components are essential for achieving predefined quality standards and meeting the study's primary objectives, covering aspects like informed consent, investigational products, primary and confirmatory secondary endpoints, critical subject safety measures, intercurrent events, key study population aspects, measures to prevent study bias, and specifics required for study submission.

QA would probably say that it will be easier to separate it into critical *processes* and critical *data* for primary objectives and Endpoints:

Examples of Critical Processes

Example 1 – Patient Recruitment and Enrollment
The process of patient recruitment and enrollment stands as a critical determinant of trial success, directly impacting the study's statistical power and validity. Delays or inadequacies in patient recruitment can compromise the study timeline and sample size, thereby jeopardizing the accuracy and reliability of trial results.

Let's take an example. In a Phase II oncology trial evaluating the efficacy of a novel immunotherapy, the timely recruitment of eligible patients within specified criteria is critical to ensuring sufficient statistical power for detecting treatment effects. Delays in patient enrollment may prolong the trial duration and increase the risk of confounding factors, potentially affecting the interpretation of treatment outcomes.

Example 2 – Data Collection and Management
The process of data collection and management serves as the backbone of clinical trial operations, underpinning the generation of reliable and

interpretable study findings. Accurate and complete data capture, coupled with robust data management practices, is imperative for maintaining data integrity and regulatory compliance throughout the trial.

A great example could be a Phase III cardiovascular trial assessing the efficacy of a new anticoagulant, for which the accurate collection and documentation of patient-reported outcomes (PROs), such as AEs and clinical endpoints (e.g., myocardial infarction, stroke), are critical to determining the drug's safety profile and efficacy. Any discrepancies or omissions in data collection may compromise the validity of trial results and regulatory submissions.

Examples of Critical Data for Primary Objectives and Endpoints

Example 1 – Primary Endpoint Measurement

The precise measurement and assessment of primary endpoints constitute a critical aspect of clinical trial conduct, directly influencing the determination of treatment efficacy and regulatory approval. Primary endpoints typically represent key clinical outcomes or endpoints that reflect the therapeutic effect of the investigational intervention.

A great example could be a Phase III diabetes trial evaluating the efficacy of a novel insulin analog. The primary endpoint may be defined as the reduction in HbA1c levels from baseline to the end of the treatment period. Accurate and standardized methods for HbA1c measurement, along with rigorous endpoint adjudication processes, are essential to ensuring the reliability and validity of treatment comparisons.

Example 2 – Critical Data Variables

Critical data variables encompass specific data points or measurements that hold paramount importance in assessing treatment effects, safety outcomes, and overall trial success. These variables are typically predefined based on clinical relevance, regulatory requirements, and study objectives.

We will take as an example a Phase II vaccine trial targeting respiratory syncytial virus (RSV) infection. Critical data variables may include the incidence of RSV-related hospitalizations, the frequency of respiratory symptoms (e.g., cough, wheezing), and the presence of RSV-specific antibodies in serum samples. These data elements serve as key indicators of vaccine efficacy and safety, guiding regulatory decision-making and clinical practice recommendations.

Quality Tolerance Limits (QTLs)

Before delving into the responsibility for this process, let's take a moment to discuss QTLs. A QTL serves to establish an acceptable threshold for critical quality attributes. It delineates the predetermined acceptable boundaries for parameters critical to quality that directly influence the safety, efficacy, and integrity of study data.

QTL helps identify and mitigate risks associated with critical processes and data in clinical trials.

By setting QTLs, organizations can establish clear thresholds for acceptable quality levels, enabling proactive risk management and ensuring compliance with regulatory requirements.

In the regulatory framework, QTLs are implicitly referenced in various guidelines and regulations governing clinical research, including ICH E6 (R2) Good Clinical Practice (GCP) guidelines and regulatory requirements from FDA and EMA. These guidelines emphasize the importance of implementing quality management systems and risk-based approaches to ensure the protection of human subjects and the reliability of clinical trial data.

Setting QTLs for a clinical trial must involve QA alongside other stakeholders. The QA representative brings unique insights and a systematic approach that are crucial for comprehensive risk assessment and management. QA's involvement ensures that the process is not only thorough but also aligned with the highest standards of quality and compliance.

Setting QTL for a Study Involves Several Steps:

1. You will not be surprised that first we need to identify the CTQs: as we described earlier, determine the key parameters or variables that directly impact the safety, efficacy, or integrity of the study data. These may include primary endpoints, key safety parameters, and critical processes. QA involvement will guarantee that QTLs are set in compliance with regulatory guidelines and based on solid scientific rationale.

2. Defining Acceptance Criteria: the specific criteria or limits for each identified CTQ should be based on scientific rationale, historical data, regulatory requirements, and clinical significance.

3. Selecting Measurement Tools: Choose appropriate measurement tools or methods to assess the identified CTQs. This may involve analytical techniques, laboratory assays, or clinical assessments.

4. Risk Assessment: Conduct a risk assessment to identify potential risks associated with each CTQ and prioritize them based on severity and likelihood of occurrence. QA's risk assessment culture brings a proactive approach to identifying and mitigating potential risks. By incorporating QA insights, the risk assessment process becomes more robust, addressing both foreseeable and unforeseen issues that could impact trial integrity.

5. Setting QTL: Based on the risk assessment and scientific evidence, determine the QTL for each CTQ, specifying the acceptable range or limits within which the data must fall to ensure patient safety and data integrity.

6. Validation and Verification: Validate the selected measurement tools and verification procedures to ensure their accuracy, reliability, and suitability for the intended purpose. QA plays a crucial role in ensuring these processes meet stringent quality standards.

Practical Examples of Setting QTLs Include:

- For a cardiovascular trial, setting QTLs for blood pressure measurements to ensure adherence to predefined thresholds for systolic and diastolic pressures.

- Establishing QTLs for laboratory parameters such as serum biomarker levels or hematological values to monitor patient health and treatment response.

- Defining QTLs for AEs or safety endpoints to identify predefined criteria for severity and frequency.

- Determining QTLs for data completeness and accuracy involving PROs. In this scenario, a QTL could be established to ensure that a certain percentage of data fields are completed for each patient visit, and that the entered data accurately reflects the patient's responses. For instance, if the study protocol requires patients to report their pain levels using a numerical rating scale (NRS), the QTL may specify that at least 90% of patients must provide valid NRS scores at each visit, with outliers flagged for review. Additionally, the QTL could define acceptable error rates for data entry and transcription to maintain data integrity throughout the study.

Setting QTLs involves collaboration between cross-functional teams, including clinical operations, data management, biostatistics, and regulatory affairs. Utilizing risk assessment tools such as Failure Mode and Effects Analysis (FMEA) or Ishikawa diagrams can help identify potential sources of variation and prioritize critical parameters for QTL determination.

QA instills a culture of continuous improvement and rigorous monitoring. This mindset ensures that QTLs are not static but are periodically reviewed and adjusted based on ongoing trial data and feedback, maintaining high standards throughout the study lifecycle.

Recognizing and embedding the role of QA in these processes is crucial for driving the cultural change needed to achieve higher standards of quality in clinical studies.

Aspects to Consider When Determining QTLs

Aspects	Why
Applicable regulatory guidance and industry standards	To identify any specific requirements or recommendations for data completeness and accuracy thresholds.
Study Objectives	Critical data elements essential for assessing safety and efficacy may require higher thresholds than less critical data.
Potential risks	To identify potential risks associated with incomplete or inaccurate data/data errors.
Historical data (from similar studies or therapeutic areas)	To understand typical rates of data completeness and accuracy by analyzing historical data.
Feasibility of threshold	To align with practical limitations coming out from the study settings.
Stakeholders Input	To gather input based on their expertise and experience.

Additional Factors to Consider

- Patient population
- Data collection methods
- Available and trained resources for data monitoring and QA

Overall, setting QTL in clinical trials is essential for ensuring the quality and integrity of study data, mitigating risks, and ultimately safeguarding patient safety and welfare.

Let's focus now on who are the key stakeholders involved in managing risks through RBQM.

- Clinical Data Managers (CDMs): CDMs, as the de facto custodians of clinical data, play a pivotal role in overseeing data quality and ensuring compliance with regulatory requirements. They are responsible for identifying potential risks, implementing risk mitigation strategies, and continuously monitoring trial data to maintain quality standards.
- Cross-functional Teams: RBQM involves collaboration among various stakeholders, including clinical operations, regulatory affairs, biostatistics, medical affairs teams, and QA teams. Cross-functional teams work together to identify risk indicators, develop risk management plans, and implement corrective actions to address identified risks.
- Sponsor: Sponsor companies hold the ultimate accountability for the conduct and outcomes of clinical trials. Even when outsourcing

these activities to CROs, which is common practice, the sponsor has to provide evidence of having maintained adequate oversight. "Adequate" includes the responsibility for establishing RBQM frameworks, providing resources and support for risk management activities, and ensuring that trial activities adhere to regulatory standards and guidelines.

The responsibility for initiating, overseeing, and sustaining this process throughout the study doesn't rest on QA but emanates from a QA-centric viewpoint. Consequently, while QA may not be explicitly listed among stakeholders, the culture of risk management holds a central role within the organizational ethos, influencing the collective perspective of all involved.

To summarize, RBQM encompasses several key components that synergistically contribute to its efficacy:

Before the Study Start

RBQM begins with a meticulous examination of trial processes, protocols, and data streams to identify potential risks. These risks may range from protocol deviations and data inaccuracies to operational inefficiencies and compliance gaps.

For example, consider a clinical trial investigating the efficacy of a new cancer drug. A risk assessment reveals a potential risk of medication errors due to complex dosing instructions. By identifying this risk upfront, the trial team can implement enhanced training protocols and dosage monitoring measures to mitigate the risk and ensure patient safety.

During the Study

Once risks are identified, they are systematically assessed and prioritized based on their severity, likelihood, and impact on trial objectives. This prioritization enables focused allocation of resources and attention to high-risk areas.

To illustrate this, let's envision a scenario where, during a risk assessment for a cardiovascular trial, the team identifies a crucial risk linked to patient non-compliance with medication regimens. By giving priority to this risk, the team devises specific patient education strategies and implements adherence monitoring protocols. As a result, the likelihood of AEs is significantly diminished.

RBQM entails the development and implementation of proactive risk mitigation strategies aimed at minimizing the likelihood and impact of identified risks. These strategies may include process improvements, training initiatives, enhanced monitoring protocols, and technological interventions.

Let's take a real-world example. In a Phase III oncology trial, the trial team identifies a significant risk of data discrepancies due to manual data entry errors. To mitigate this risk, the team implements EDC systems with built-in validation checks and real-time data monitoring capabilities, ensuring data accuracy and integrity throughout the trial.

RBQM emphasizes the importance of ongoing monitoring and adaptation to evolving risks throughout the trial lifecycle. Continuous data review, trend analysis, and feedback mechanisms enable timely detection of emerging risks and prompt adjustment of mitigation strategies.

Practical Tip: implement regular risk review meetings involving cross-functional stakeholders to discuss emerging risks, assess the effectiveness of mitigation measures, and adapt strategies as needed. The documentation of these meetings and the actions taken as a result of the implemented RBQM plan will go a long way in an audit from a regulatory agency.

After the Study

Well, now it is too late!

Unfortunately, there are still so many examples coming across my desk or shared with me by colleagues, where start-up timelines, resource pressures during the study conduct, or a certain degree of inexperience caused the omission of implementing and executing an adequate and proactive RBQM plan.

Having said this, we have to acknowledge that despite the best intentions, no RBQM plan is going to be perfect, and quality/data issues might only be detected after the fact. In this case, rigorous transparency around the timing, scope, and nature of the scope needs to be documented, including information on how these findings might impact the interpretation of the study, how corrections, if applicable, will be conducted, and how this gap will be prevented from happening in the future.

Risk-Based Quality Management – What Risks? Who Manages?

Within clinical research, the role of CDM has been interpreted differently for a long time. Those organizations, regardless of representing a sponsor, CRO, or technology company, who have managed to position CDM at the center of the overall clinical trial delivery, have been considered the progressive winners of the game.

Without trustworthy clinical data as a tangible outcome, best planned and executed clinical trials do not bring any value to anyone who has been involved and who has invested time and budget; first and foremost, we fall short of delivering for the patients who are waiting for improved treatment options.

For sure, good quality of clinical data has always been one of the main topics to consider in the journey to answer clinical study specific questions, by creating scientific evidence to answer those questions.

There have always been considerations on how to mitigate the risk related to data quality. In fact, the management of clinical data started as a rather retractive effort to identify issues and address them after they had occurred. With this retrospective approach, assessing and managing the quality of clinical data also resides in the past, which as we all know cannot be changed anymore.

This is one of the reasons why RBQM is playing an ever-increasing role here and now and is directly correlated to the evolution of CDM leading RBQM and moving the needle toward a proactive mindset.

Let us start with an understanding of "What are the fundamental building blocks of RBQM?"

At this stage, we have already established CDM's main role and reason for our existence. CDM has always been devoted to performing good clinical trials. Well, don't we all? And how do you define a good clinical study?

I hope we can all agree on the fact that when we deliver true and trustworthy answers to scientific questions, respect participants' rights, and run the most efficient possible study, we will have done a good job for the patient, the industry, and the advancement of knowledge. And, if we focus for a moment on RBQM's contribution to the desired outcome, we can surely agree as well on the paramount importance it carries toward achieving this goal. This requires a change in our way of thinking about clinical data quality, by asking questions such as:

- Is the ultimate quality of clinical data an error-free state?
- Can this be achieved and has this ever been achieved?
- Would it be sufficient if we were to solely focus on possible errors related to primary and secondary endpoints, as well as patients' safety?
- How do we establish a new "quality balance" or a new norm for what is acceptable quality and where can we find reliable guidance?

Both regulators, the FDA and the EMA, have clarified their position with the publication of respective guidance in 2013. For example, the US Department of Health and Human Services, through its FDA-operating division, suggested that 100% SDV only provides minimal benefit and recommended focusing instead on critical data points for a sample of subjects and study visits as an indicator of data accuracy.

They also noted that SDV of noncritical data may not provide significantly useful information to the sponsor, since errors do not affect the outcome of the trial (Source: Sheetz, Nicole et al. "Evaluating Source Data Verification as a Quality Control Measure in Clinical Trials" – TransCelerate, 2014).

The EMA also contributed to the topic by outlining that current practices in clinical research are not proportionate to risk. They suggested that the problem may stem from an overinterpretation or misunderstanding of regulatory environment or a failure to evolve processes and resistance to new approaches, for example, application of single model monitoring for all trials, which is neither appropriate nor effective.

In summary the Health Authority recommendations are creating two key areas of focus:

1) On critical data elements, for example,

- Patient Safety
- Primary Endpoints
- Secondary Endpoints

2) Focus on "Errors that matter"

In combination, these re-focused activities targeting clinical data quality are using more data surveillance methods based on centralized statistical monitoring.

The new clinical monitoring paradigm requires that each study team conducts a robust risk assessment and identify study-specific risks that can be mitigated through monitoring intervention. In addition, to be specific, it means applying critical thinking and not a one-size-fits-all approach. The ask is clear; specify risks a priori at the start of the study and also consider those risks which can arise over the course of a study, and which can be

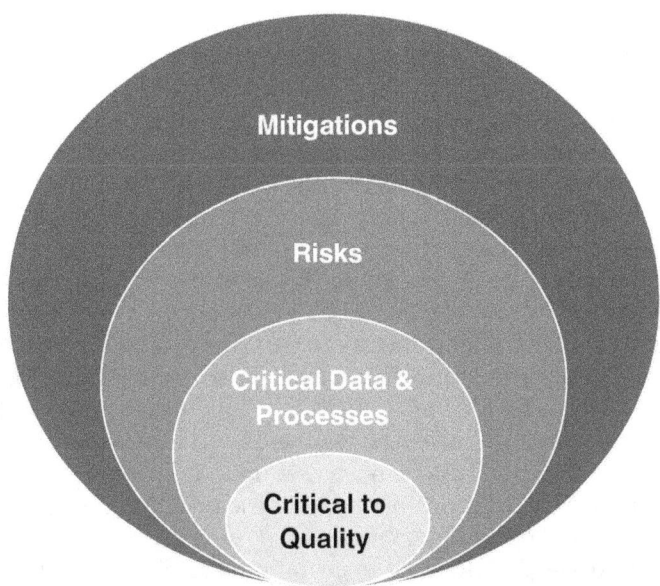

FIGURE 3.1
New Clinical Monitoring Paradigm.

either prevented or managed through pro-active measures to prevent their occurrence.

Following the philosophy of "Know your risks", we need to ensure that the monitoring strategies are tailored to risks that are focused on Critical Data and Processes. Under Critical Data we understand the data that are critical to the reliability of the study findings, specifically those data that support primary and secondary endpoints, as well as data that relates to subject safety and rights. For Critical Processes, there is a general understanding that it refers to those processes that deal with items related to the reliability of the study findings, and, again, to those related to ensuring patients' safety and rights' protection.

Changing the focus of the monitoring and evaluation of the clinical data quality requires different skills; therefore, Risk Management Roles need to be involved at the early stage of the clinical study planning and throughout the course of the study.

These roles are accountable for applying a risk-based approach to quality management that focuses on critical data and processes and monitor risk assessments to ensure adequate protection of the rights, welfare, and safety of the participants, as well as quality and integrity of the data provided by the clinical sites and all other data sources.

The FDA and EMA guidance was followed by the release of the ICH GCP E6 (R2) in 2016 and ICH GCP E6 (R3) at the beginning of 2025, in which we have been encouraged to further evolve our understanding of RBM and, consequently, connect it to the overall data review activities. Despite the release of the new guidance, many of us were having difficulties in actually implementing new processes to support the future vision of a risk-based approach.

Between 2017 and 2018 many sponsors moved toward an IDRP and many CROs have been offering such plans to support other sponsors in implementing these plans and ensuring compliance. The IDRP has become a cross-functional agreement to describe the comprehensive data review to be conducted remotely by each data reviewer, such as Clinical Data Manager and medical monitor. The study site monitor or CRA role in this process was to connect the remote data review with the on-site activities, such as Source Data Validation (SDV) or Review (SDR) or supporting the sites to answer queries. With the IDRP and its intention to ensure a holistic centralized data review plan of all accumulating data, we have also committed to focus on the defined critical data. The defined critical data not only drives the data review activities by each role but also defines the SDV that will be performed by the Site Monitor in EDC. This plan was set up to ensure mutual exclusivity across data reviewers, in coordination with the programmed edit checks in the EDC system and clinical database.

A big step forward! And a big expectation, too. Starting with the same or very similar understanding of clinical data quality, functional areas touching the clinical data working hand in hand, and preventing multiplications of data validation efforts, and finally supporting the study sites by reducing their burden related to same or similar queries asked by many functions.

While many organizations have invested significant efforts into the change management driving the RBM, in many cases this paradigm change has generally been misunderstood as an SDV reduction and associated primary with site monitoring cost reduction. At least since the TransCelerate-sponsored article (Therapeutic Innovation & Regulatory Science 2014, Vol. 48(6) 671–680 "Evaluating Source Data Verification as a Quality Control Measure in Clinical Research"), based on a rigorous analysis of the 100% SDV impact on data quality, we have been provided evidence that SDV only impacted 1% (!) of the eCRF data on average. It needs to be pointed out at this stage this 1% of data is responsible for one of the biggest cost factors of clinical studies overall.

Sponsors' and service providers' adherence to the traditional way of managing the sites, with the illusion of increasing data quality through 100% SDV, has been changing very slowly. There is no evidence in publications or industry exchange forums that the few companies who decided to drastically reduce SDV which is the point-to-point comparison of data from health records with entries, say, in electronic Case Report From (eCRF) have been reporting more critical or major inspections findings on their studies than those who stayed at the high level of SDV.

Based on a pilot study with reduced SDV combined with deployment of RBM, where the on-site monitoring frequency decreased as the study progressed, a subsequent inspection conducted by the Pharmaceutical and Medical Devices Agency found no significant nonconformance that would have affected the study results and patient safety. This confirmed the prevailing industry sentiment to continue to grow RBM adoption (Higa, A., Yagi, M., Hayashi, K. et al. Risk-Based Monitoring Approach to Ensure the Quality of Clinical Study Data and Enable Effective Monitoring. Ther Innov Regul Sci 54, 139–143 (2020)).

The second component of the source data management process beside the SDV, the SDR – which is the check if the health records data is plausible, complete, consistent, and meaningful in context of patient-level study activities – has been considered as the meaningful way to ensure the right level for quality and integrity of data and support higher quality of critical data elements that <u>cannot</u> be checked by remote methods of monitoring patients' safety and data integrity. RBM implementation at the study level was triggering the evolution of the Site Monitoring activities and the consensus to focus on the errors that matter was leading to targeted SDV/SDR tailored to the most important data and processes for the study. Consequently, on-site monitoring became the area to develop and maintain trusted communication with the sites, and the CRAs had the chance to utilize the off-site monitoring by using output of Centralized Monitoring to discuss with sites the data completeness, outliers, trends, and signals. With this the site and data monitoring areas have been also structured to an inter-connected approach to look at the data in a holistic way.

TransCelerate's RBM guide has been paying attention to a modernized, proactive method of clinical trial monitoring and an adaptive approach directing monitoring toward the activities in the evolving areas with the most potential to impact patient safety and data quality. The best results can be expected when the study-specific monitoring strategy, built upon the study-specific risk assessment, unifies in the prospective monitoring methods to a comprehensive picture of RBM execution, as presented by TransCelerate.

On a practical level this means that the three areas of monitoring, that is, centralized, on-site, and off-site, can and should be planned for and executed in such a way to not duplicate efforts from a clinical operation point of view, and most importantly, use CDM insights and RBQM outputs to guide all monitoring activities.

Study types, phases, therapeutic areas, and primary/secondary endpoints should guide the required extent of each monitoring tool in hand. The RBM approach needs to be in-sync with the data review and RBQM plan put in place for a given study. On an operational level, this means that the functional areas of Clinical Operations and CDM must work closely together as equal partners toward the common goal of adequate monitoring.

All parts of the RBQM implementation at the study level have an integral role in controlling the study risks. Focusing on the data quality (from GCP Guidance ICH E6 (R2) 2016, Section 5.18.3):

> Centralized monitoring is a remote evaluation of accumulating data, performed in a timely manner, supported by appropriately qualified and trained persons (e.g., data managers, biostatisticians). Centralized monitoring processes provide additional monitoring capabilities that can complement and reduce the extent and/or frequency of on-site monitoring and help distinguish between reliable data and potentially unreliable data.

Review, which may include statistical analyses, of accumulating data from centralized monitoring, can be used to identify:

- Missing data
- Inconsistent data
- Data outliers
- Unexpected lack of variability
- Protocol deviations
- Cross-site variability trends
- Systematic and/or significant errors in data collection and reporting by site or across sites
- Potential data manipulation
- Data integrity problems

Knowing this book is all about CDM and looking at the list above with Clinical Data as a leading part, the next logical step is to consider Centralized Monitoring as an extension of CDM. This is a paradigm shift. This is a new mindset. An evolutionary step for CDM.

Site Monitoring is still an integral part of the RBM Methodology using the RBQM tools created within this area for flexible translation toward the frequency of monitoring activities.

QTL levels set at study start related to areas such as Data Collection, Protocol Deviations, and AEs reporting, together with Key Risk Indicators (KRIs), will respectively increase on-site monitoring in case of detected risks via these QTLs and KRIs.

Appropriate mitigations identified through the aforementioned assessments must be included in the Monitoring Plan and adhered to cross-functionally as the study evolves.

The COVID-19 pandemic had the positive impact of accelerating the implementation of RBM methodologies end to end, meaning not only the consideration of reducing SDV but also how to better use inflowing clinical data through centralized monitoring to ensure patient safety and data integrity.

"The Risk-Based Quality Management Concept is the whole system not just the last component of monitoring!" This is how the FDA's Director David Burrow began his speech on July 17, 2019, in the Robert J. Margolis Center for Health Policy at Duke University (Home | Margolis Institute for Health Policy (duke.edu) https://healthpolicy.duke.edu/).

What Is the Difference Between RBM and RBQM?

- RBM written into US/EU regulations in 2013 mandated the sponsors to use technology and real-time information to proactively monitor risk and support critical thinking and decision-making process via the ability to identify and correct issues as and when they arise.

- RBQM applies the principles of RBM to all areas of quality management including the shift to use of electronic and digital technologies (EDC, ePRO, IRT) and the transition from paper-based data collection.

- RBQM encompasses all elements of the study, from planning right through to execution. Risk management underpins the overall quality of the trial by identifying, controlling, and communicating the risks AND through implementation and utilization of an effective centralized monitoring approach.

From my perspective this evolution from RBM to RBQM is not only a tremendous opportunity to plan and manage clinical research more effectively and efficiently in the environment of growing research complexity, duration, and cost.

With clinical data as an ultimate source driving all the RBQM activities, it is the birth of a new era for CDM. It is the switch between the time when we have been running after the issues which have happened in the past, to a world where we utilize clinical data to predict the future and prevent the errors from happening in the first place.

How Do We Enable Improved Clinical Data Quality?

Here is a sample of some truly striking passages of the respective guidelines not only supporting the case for a "data quality first" mentality but also eliminating waste of time and resources on non-critical-to-success-data.

ICH GCP E6 R2

Quality Management (Sponsor)

The sponsor should implement a system to manage quality throughout all stages of the trial process. Sponsors should focus on trial activities essential to ensuring human subject protection and the reliability of trial results. Quality management includes the design of efficient clinical trial protocols, tools, and procedures for data collection and processing, as well as the collection of information that is essential to decision-making. The methods used to assure and control the quality of the trial should be proportionate to the risks inherent in the trial and the importance of the information collected. The sponsor should ensure that all aspects of the trial are operationally feasible and should avoid unnecessary complexity, procedures, and data collection. Protocols, case report forms, and other operational documents should be clear, concise, and consistent.

(A Risk-Based Approach to Monitoring of Clinical Investigations-Questions and Answers (fda.gov) – April 2023)

As described in the 2013 RBM guidance, FDA recommends that at the protocol design stage, sponsors identify the critical data and processes necessary for human subject protection and maintaining data integrity for the investigation. Once these are identified, sponsors should perform a risk assessment and determine whether possible risks to critical data and processes have to be defined and monitored throughout the study.

ICH GCP E6 R3

And in terms of latest releases and likely the most powerful one, we have ICH E6 (R3) since the beginning of 2025. A link to an explanatory video as well as some of the key passages are given below. A breakthrough for CDM is section 4 of this guideline, which many, including myself, see as a direct call for action for CDM leadership in the pursuit of data integrity.

ICH E6 R3 Explanatory Video:
database.ich.org/sites/default/files/ICH_E6%28R3%29_Guideline_GCP_Video_2023_0601.mp4

Data and Records

Data Handling

The sponsor should ensure the integrity and confidentiality of data generated and managed.

The sponsor should apply quality control to the relevant stages of data handling to ensure that the data are of sufficient quality to generate reliable results. The sponsor should focus their QA and quality control activities and data review on critical data, including its relevant metadata.

The sponsor should ensure that documented processes are implemented to ensure the data integrity for the full data life cycle.

Review of Data and Metadata

Procedures for review of trial-specific data, audit trails, and other relevant metadata should be in place. It should be a planned activity, and the extent and nature should be risk-based, adapted to the individual trial, and adjusted based on experience during the trial.

ICH GCP E8 R1

Lastly, we come to ICH GCP E8 (R1), which also emphasizes in some sections the guidance of focusing on what is truly important, or to use the regulatory words, the "critical to quality factors". Some of the relevant passages are these:

Designing Quality Into Clinical Studies

The quality by design approach to clinical research (Section 3.1 in the guideline) involves focusing on CTQ factors to ensure the protection of the rights, safety, and wellbeing of study participants; the generation of reliable and meaningful results; and the management of risks to those factors using a risk-proportionate approach (Section 3.2 in the guideline). The approach is supported by the establishment of an appropriate framework for the identification and review of CTQ factors (Section 3.3 in the guideline) at the time of design and planning of the study, and throughout its conduct, analysis, and reporting.

CTQ Factors

A basic set of factors relevant to ensuring study quality should be identified for each study. Emphasis should be given to those factors that stand out as critical to study quality. These CTQ factors are attributes of a study whose integrity is fundamental to the protection of study participants, the reliability and interpretability of the study results, and the decisions made based on the study results. These quality factors are considered to be critical because, if their integrity were to be undermined by errors of design or conduct, the reliability or ethics of decision-making based on the results of the study would also be undermined. CTQ factors should also be considered holistically, so that dependencies among them can be identified. Section 7 of this document provides considerations that can help identify CTQ factors for a study.

Considerations in Identifying CTQ Factors

The identification of CTQ factors should be supported by proactive, cross-functional discussions and decision-making at the time of study planning, as described in Section 3. Different factors will stand out as critical for different types of studies, following the concepts introduced in Sections 4 through 6.

In designing a study, the following aspects should be considered, where applicable, to support the identification of CTQ factors:

- Engagement of all relevant stakeholders, including patients, is considered during study planning and design.

To answer the data quality question, regulators are encouraging us to apply critical thinking and start at the planning stage of the clinical trial by defining fit for purpose and reliable information to address the key questions in decision-making process.

The first step is to define the CTQ factors which are those aspects of study design or conduct critical to impact the following:

- Protection of study subjects
- Generating reliable data
- Decisions made based on the study results

Following the CTQ factors, an assessment to identify study-specific risks is needed. Some of the risks may be accepted, but those which can be mitigated through monitoring intervention will impact the next steps.

Such information is the basis to build quality into the study protocol and processes, resulting in Quality by Design (QbD), where we focus on:

- CTQ factors to ensure protection of study subjects and data reliability
- Proper management of the risks to the CTQ factors (e.g., by implementing a risk-based quality management system)

Based on the nature of the study-specific risks to be mitigated and the clinical trial design, the monitoring activities combining the site monitoring (performed on-site or remotely) and centralized monitoring need to be defined to a study-specific monitoring strategy. According to ICH E6 R3 section 3.11.4, the sponsor should determine the appropriate extent and nature of monitoring, based on identified risks.

The Case for CDM's Lead Role in RBQM

CDMs are uniquely positioned to spearhead RBQM initiatives due to their comprehensive understanding of clinical trial data and processes. The risk management culture and risk-based approach, emanating from the QA perspective, profoundly impacts the CDM role. Much of the knowledge CDMs acquire is influenced by QA impact and culture within a company. For instance, in decision junctions around the RBQM process, the involvement of QA in CDM work could significantly benefit.

Consider a scenario where a CDM is tasked with identifying potential risks to data integrity in a clinical trial. With guidance from QA-driven risk management practices, CDM can effectively assess data quality and implement robust validation strategies. This proactive approach not only ensures data integrity but also enhances patient safety. By leveraging risk assessment tools and methodologies prioritized through a QA lens, CDM can mitigate risks early in the trial lifecycle, minimizing potential disruptions and safeguarding trial outcomes.

Furthermore, CDMs' compliance knowledge, honed through QA-driven practices, ensures adherence to regulatory requirements and industry standards. By integrating QA principles into their work, CDMs uphold the integrity of trial activities, mitigating compliance-related risks and contributing to the overall success of RBQM initiatives.

In challenging the undervalued perception of the CDM role, it's essential to recognize the extensive requirements and vast knowledge it entails, shaped significantly by organization culture.

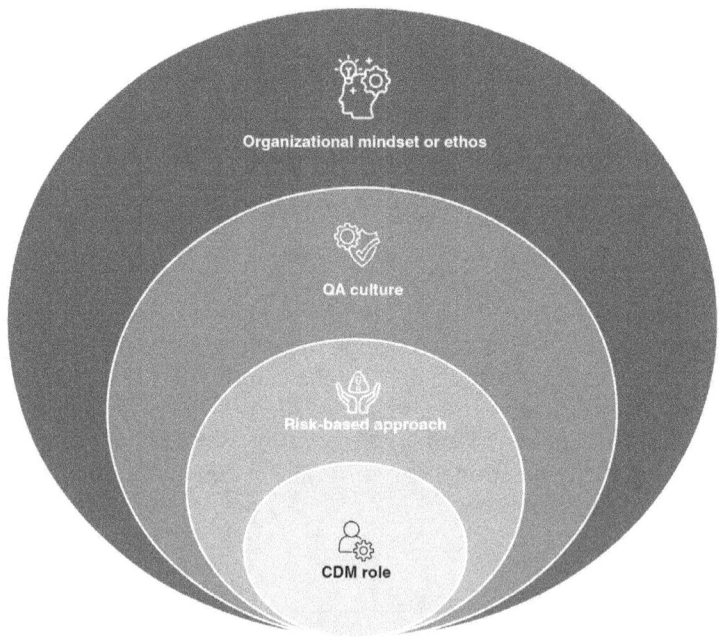

FIGURE 3.2
Eye of the tiger: CDM's role is influenced by the environment that surrounds it.

Defining CTQ factors requires cross-functional alignment at the study level, and the functions owning the clinical data like Statisticians and Clinical Data Mangers provide key information in this decision-making process.

On the CTQ basis Critical Data and Processes (CD&P) are derived as translational step toward the main areas of the clinical trial execution:

- Risk Management (RM)
- Centralized Monitoring (CM)
- Clinical Data (CD)
- Clinical Vendors (CV)

For each of those areas the CTQ factors and the CD&P are the same and all functions are working toward the best results in translating them to their areas of competencies.

Risk Management personnel will use them for the study-specific risk-driven prioritization and reprioritization of risk oversight and effectiveness check, which include execution of mitigation implementation (i.e. ensuring that identified risks are being addressed until full resolution).

Centralized Monitoring CD&P translation of study-specific requirements leads into Data Quality Strategy reflected in the Centralized Monitoring Plan, which connects area-specific Key Risk Indicators (KRIs) and QTLs for CDM, Monitoring, and Vendor Management teams. Many examples of the previously mentioned IDRP evolved into some form of Integrated Data *Quality Review Plan* and by doing so directly connecting Centralized Monitoring to CDM.

CDM, when not already the function leading Centralized Monitoring, is one of the main contributors to the study-specific risk assessment and the key player in executing the Centralized Monitoring plan. The dedicated CD&P translation leads to a focused or targeted data review, where the data presence and data sense types of checks are not spread equally across all data as this has been done in the past, but *CTQ-driven Clinical Data Quality Oversight* is being additionally supported by CM tools like with CDM KRIs or QTLs. The Clinical Data Manager must also contribute and ideally lead the risk assessment and the mitigation of some of the risks associated with CTQ factors. The Risk Assessment must go beyond the typical risks impacting study timelines, deviation from data standards, or identifying critical data and processes. (The adoption of risk-based CDM approaches (Version #1) SCDM Innovation Committee – CDS Topic Brief Version 1 [July 2022]).

With an increasing amount of data coming from outside of the EDC systems and being delivered by a high range of clinical data vendors, this area could be considered with a separate set of CD&P translations closely connected to the outcome of Vendor Risk Assessment and Management and Data Quality Oversight with specific KPIs as well.

CDM has a huge potential to include the Centralized Monitoring, based on the fact that both functional areas are based on clinical data to manage the quality and translate the specific requirements into *Data Quality Strategy*.

In a model of connected functional areas the clinical data validation and oversight are interconnected by KRIs, CM Signals, QTLs, data issues, and diversified monitoring activities. Ideally the data is then validated in connection with all involved functional areas' activities holistically, and the number of queries, especially those considered duplicates asked separately by specific functions, is eliminated or at least decreasing drastically.

From "One-Size-Fits-All" to Risk-Proportionate Data Quality Approach

The involvement of the CDM at each stage of the clinical trial has changed over time and continues to change as the RBQM implementation is accelerating this evolution significantly. CDM must keep up this significant expansion of role from the legacy of QC-based strategies if it is to support QbD by 1) identifying CTQ factors, 2) de-risking the protocol, and 3) performing a CDM-specific risk assessment. Only then can CDM implement safe and effective risk-based study execution strategies paired with robust continuous process improvements to deliver quality data sufficient to support good decision-making. This will have a dramatic impact on the CDM roles by moving from catching mistakes to identifying problems that may jeopardize

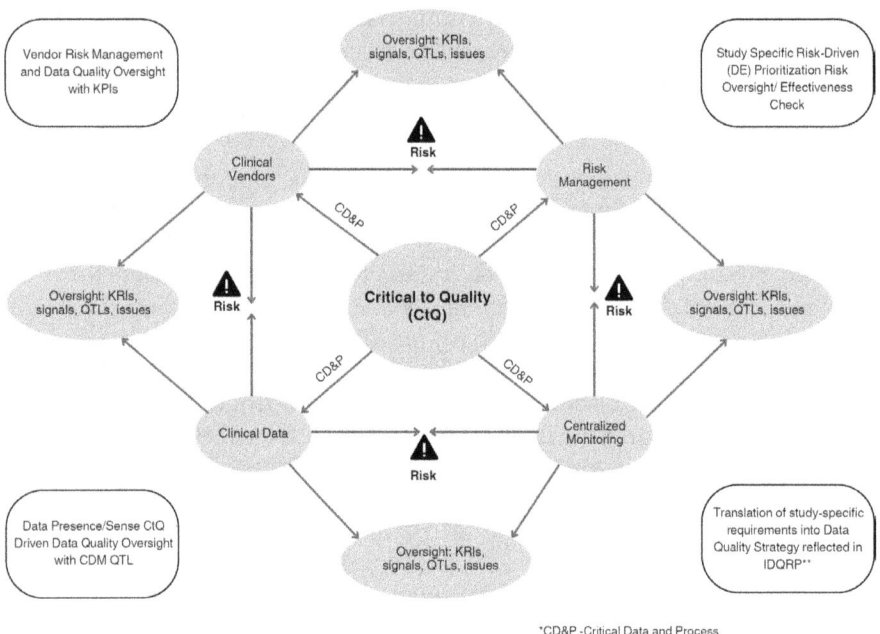

FIGURE 3.3
Risk-Proportionate Data Quality Approach.

the trial. Overall, the end-to-end management of the operational and scientific risks shown below must be embedded throughout the entire CDM Framework, with connection to other functions involved in the process when necessary. (The adoption of risk-based CDM approaches (Version #1) SCDM Innovation Committee – CDS Topic Brief Version 1 [July 2022].)

With changing CDM processes to Risk-Based Data Quality Management, where the CDM involvement is generally changing toward proactive data risk and issue managers, there is a need to up-skill the profiles and extend the areas of interest. Not only do we need CDM risk managers in the way of such evolution, but we also need new roles like Data Visualization Expert, with the ability to build data visualization as a graphical representation of information and data and analyze the output to receive new quality of data validation. More technical roles specialized in building the connection between the Centralized Monitoring technologies and diversity of incoming data analyzed in this environment through KPIs or QTLs. Within the Centralized Monitoring but also outside of its Machine Learning or Deep Learning Specialist will be leveraging technologies with capabilities to understand complex data and also text, as well as aspects of statistical and programming methodologies or model training and testing. New emerging CDM-related roles will be able to support risk-based data quality management with the

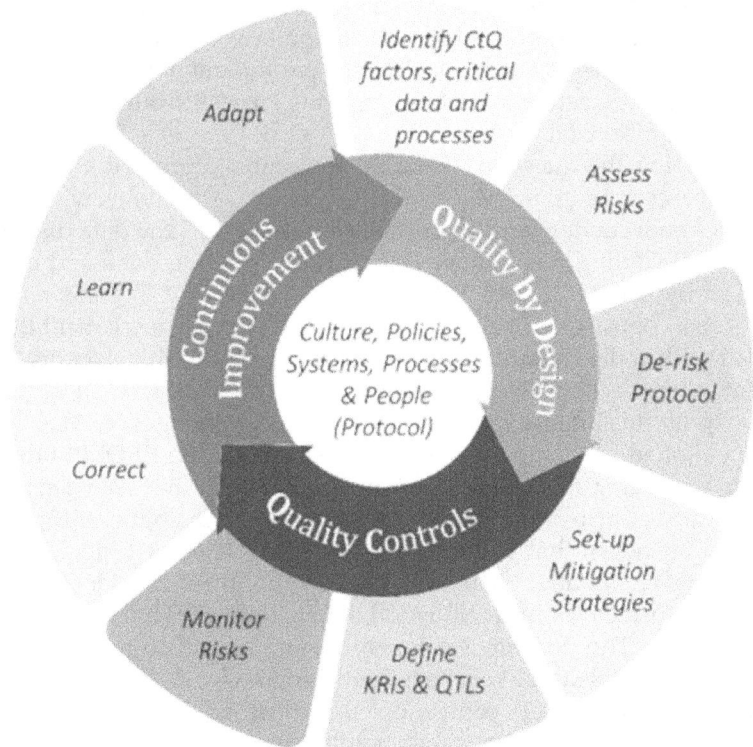

FIGURE 3.4
RBQM wheel.

switch to proactive activities supporting data risk mitigations but also predictive risk as an outcome from large volumes of data insights using state-of-the-art (AI-powered) analytics tools. This will be an opportunity to move the need toward discovering meaningful insights that have been undetectable thus far for us.

Considering the increasing vendor data, we will need roles with ability to perform huge amount of data integrations from traditional and new types of data sources like wearable devices using sensors.

Speaking about the RBQM-driven CDM evolution, we need to take into consideration the impact of new technologies, especially in relation to the EMA Guideline on computerized systems (Guideline on computerized systems and electronic data in clinical trials https://www.ema.europa.eu/en/documents/regulatory-procedural-guideline/guideline-computerised-systems-and-electronic-data-clinical-trials_en.pdf), as well as the new Section 4 (electronic data in clinical trials Data Governance ICH GCP E6 R3 Step 2b (europa.eu) https://www.ema.europa.eu/en/documents/scientific-guideline/draft-ich-e6-r3-guideline-good-clinical-practice-gcp-step-2b_en.pdf).

The risk-proportionate approach should be applied also toward the aspects of the security and validation of computerized systems and data life-cycle and user management supporting the paramount of patient safety and reliable data in sufficient quality to support the answer to our scientific questions in the clinical trial.

In answering the question "How do we enable improved clinical data quality" we cannot miss the *Effective Centralized Monitoring* with all the cross-functional connections. CDM will share with CM the data discrepancies, Medical Coding, Laboratory Data Review, missing data, and queries, but linked by RBQM in Data Management to focus on CTQ and resulting in better risk control. Medical and Safety data reviews using Patient Profiles provided within the Centralized Monitoring will make this data visible for other functions participating in CM.

To wrap up this intense dive into RBQM, a quick thought on AI.

As mentioned in the previous chapter, AI can elevate RBQM to the next level. Imagine being able to leverage the combined data and knowledge from a vast amount of historical clinical studies to determine optimal thresholds for critical elements; that is, the RBQM process, based on calculated risk, will deepen its foundation extremely. AI could use these considerations, risk management principles, and real-world data to define QTLs based on extensive knowledge. This concept is compelling, and a certified threshold determined through AI would likely be in high demand.

However, within the QA context discussed earlier, AI has its limitations. The reliability of AI-generated data is questionable. Are the information sources reliable? Can the thresholds be trusted? This raises the crucial question: how do we validate the AI-produced information?

To ensure data reliability in AI validation for our industry, robust mitigations are necessary. Maintain comprehensive records of data provenance and rigorously vet sources. Implement data cleaning procedures and conduct regular audits to ensure data quality. Cross-reference data with multiple sources and historical datasets to validate accuracy. Enforce strict access controls and maintain audit trails to secure data integrity. Conduct periodic data reviews and revalidation to keep data current. Train staff on data QA and regularly assess their competence. Develop a risk management plan and promote continuous improvement. Use third-party services for independent verification and conduct external audits. These measures enhance data integrity and ensure compliance with regulatory standards.

Given these extensive requirements, a pertinent question arises: isn't the effort required to validate AI data sources and properly teach the system far greater than implementing a risk management process that integrates all stakeholders, as described in this chapter?

Those questions are the challenges to be resolved.

Summary

This was an intense chapter where we put together the gathered knowledge of the already established pivotal role of CDM together with one of the most important examples of how to use the power of clinical data – RBQM.

We have given a detailed overview of the evolution of the global regulatory framework over the last 10+ years, providing the industry with a clear mandate to move on from the traditional SDV-focused approaches to the more advanced concept of proactive implementation of RBQM.

The need for CDM to step up our game and embrace this opportunity is not only a self-serving exercise, but overdue to complete the paradigm shift from reacting to data quality issues after they happened to a proactive mindset that will allow us to prevent many of these errors to happen at all, and thereby make patients safer, clinical studies more efficient, and our results more reliable.

4

Technology Overload – How to
Avoid Common Pitfalls

With Zia Haque

CDM technologies have evolved significantly over the past few decades. The advancements present opportunities and challenges to clinical research study teams in selecting fit-for purpose technology solutions for each study. This chapter aims to provide guidelines for teams to select appropriate CDM solutions for their studies. This chapter is divided into the following three sub chapters:

- Background and present landscape
- Technology considerations during the three phases of a clinical trial
- Supporting technology solutions

Background

Technological advancements over the past decade have enabled enhancements within the clinical research space. While it took the clinical research industry quite a while to transition from a paper-based model to EDC settings, subsequent adoption of technologies in the industry has been swifter.

Advances in direct-to-patient data collection modalities have opened vast opportunities to collect real-time data from study participants in clinical trials. These advances align well with the growing number of subject-reported data points contributing to primary study protocol aims. Direct data collection from subjects earlier on was mostly ancillary to data collected during subject visits. With growing emphasis, regulatory authorities expect subject-reported data to be reported with the same level of rigor as data collected during subject visits if these data points contribute to the study analyses.

80

DOI: 10.1201/9781003648314-4

Additional data streams such as subject voice recordings, cognitive test results, and biomarker tests have further enhanced opportunities for data collection.

Present Landscape

The common present-day practice is for teams to discuss technology solutions at a study level. Decisions related to choice of data collection platform, subject-reported data modalities, and external data streams are often hurried choices. Since the data management team is busy developing database specifications for the data collection platform, the level of scrutiny toward the other data collection streams lacks appropriate discussion to ensure all the data collection modalities can function in unison. This chapter will break down the data collection topic into three sections – start-up, conduct, and close-out – and describe the challenges and proposed solutions during each of the three phases.

Before we dive into technology challenges and solutions, let us review the following important considerations:

- Choosing fit-for-purpose technology solutions
- EDC decision tree
- Integrating external vendor data
- Qualifying vendors and vendor management
- ePRO implementation approach

Choosing Fit-For-Purpose Technology Solutions

The choice of technology solutions is paramount on all clinical research investigations. Making technology solutions in isolation, without consideration to protocol-specific nuances, will lead to misaligned technical solutions.

A decision tree to guide study teams to the most appropriate technology solutions will ensure a smooth end user experience at the study site level, while assuring data stability from the study.

Integrating External Vendor Data – To Integrate or Not?

With growing acceptance of clinical data directly from the source – the patient, the ability to harness additional types of data is ever increasing. The ability to collect real-time data from subjects in clinical trials has opened many possibilities about including these data as primary end points for

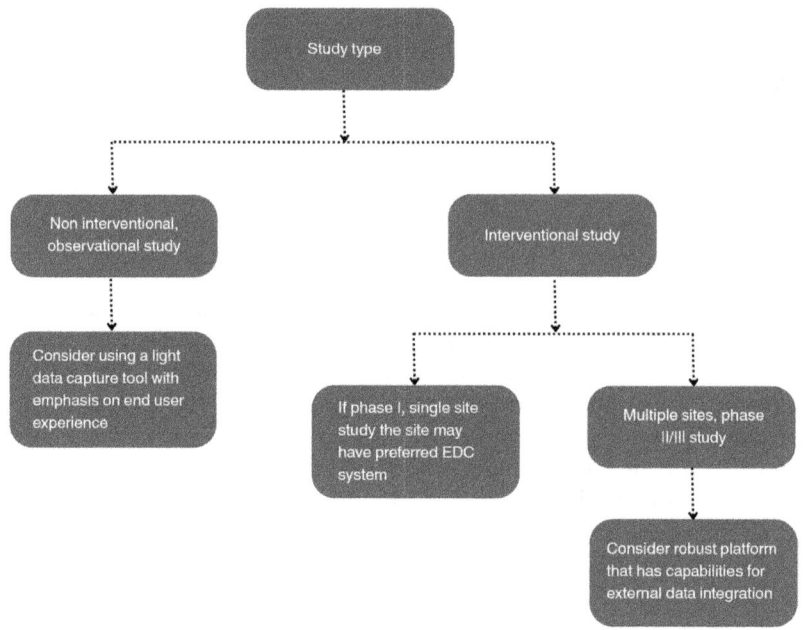

FIGURE 4.1
Decision Tree Example.

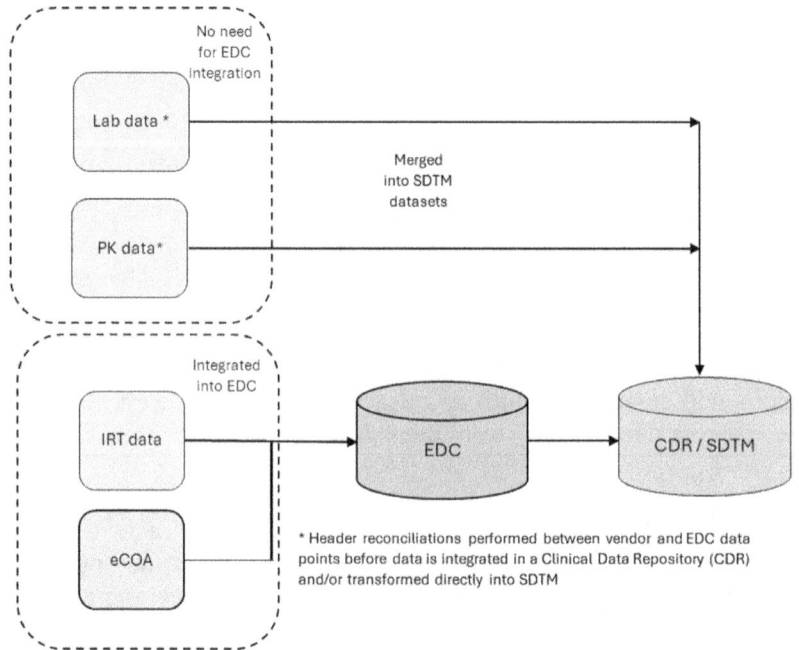

FIGURE 4.2
Data Integration Flow Example.

analyses. Regulatory authorities expect direct-to-patient data to be part of the overall data submission. Study teams should determine if there is a need to integrate data from external data sources (direct from patient data collection, external vendor data) into EDC. If integration is required, a data flow should be created to map the data streams that integrate into EDC. This will be helpful in establishing start-up timelines for the data collection technology solution to be in production ahead of first subject first visit.

Qualifying Vendors and Vendor Management

Vendor qualifying and vendor management are important considerations to ensure smooth progress during study start-up, conduct, and study close-out phases. The following aspects should be factored into the vendor qualifying and vendor management process:

- Platform capabilities including metrics reports
- Schedule regular governance meetings with vendors
- Platform roadmap
- Standard timelines for EDC build
- QA audit to assess platform-level validation
- Platform capabilities to integrate external data streams
- Integrated platform offerings – for example, IRT, eCOA
- Lead time to achieve a fully executed contract so that study start-up can proceed

It is important to set clear expectations with external data vendors and include appropriate Service-Level Agreements (SLAs) in the vendor contracts. The following aspects should be considered in the vendor management process:

- Lead time to establish Data Transfer Agreements (DTAs)
- Ensure vendors perform quality checks ahead of data transfers
- Establish turn-round times for transferring updated data transfers
- Alert vendors ahead of database locks to ensure they can send updated data transfers on time for database locks

Vendors should be audited and requalified at periodic intervals. This practice will ensure any audit findings are addressed appropriately by the vendors via CAPAs, process improvements, and SOP updates.

ePRO Implementation Approach

Over the years advances in direct-to-patient technology have identified multiple opportunities to include subject-reported data as primary data points in the study analyses. The following challenges and solutions are listed for ePRO implementation:

Gap	Solution/s
Delays in identifying appropriate ePRO scales	Ensure cross-functional team participation to select appropriate ePRO scales
Availability of appropriate eCOA for subjects during study	Cross-functional teams should participate in the ePRO UAT
Late awareness of eCOA compliance	Ensure real-time eCOA compliance reports are available, and are being reviewed on an ongoing basis to review compliance
Concerns with eCOA data quality	Review eCOA audit trial in real time to identify trends in eCOA completion. This will assist in alerting sites to retrain subjects as needed

With this background let us now look into specific technology consideration during the start-up, conduct, and close-out phases of a clinical study.

Start-up Phase

Challenges: Study teams typically become aware of a study when the start-up phase is about to begin. Technology discussions often take a back seat to other study considerations, and the theme continues during the Request for Proposal (RFP) and bid defense steps. This approach leads to decisions around data collection modalities being made in a vacuum by the data management team, with minimal to no input from stakeholders in clinical, statistical programming, and biostatistics teams. Lack of clarity on which external data streams (subject-reported data, external vendor data) need to be integrated directly into the data collection platform as opposed to being merged into the SDTM datasets may lead to delays with the study start-up process. CDM – including the study lead and the oversight role – has an important opportunity for the study's Project Manager to ensure cross-functional team review and input at this early stage. Finally, nebulousness around timelines for the data collection platform, as well as associated data streams that need to be integrated into the data collection platform being ready ahead of first subject visit, can lead to misaligned expectations within the study team. This can have an impact on starting study enrollment.

Solutions: While each study design is unique, there are proven best practices that can be applied during study start-up, regardless of the study phase or therapeutic area being investigated. The following considerations are listed as reference topics to assist teams in ensuring a smooth start in creating data collection solutions:

- Ensure awareness of pipeline among study teams to enable early engagement.

- Schedule early engagement meetings with relevant operational teams to start discussion on study design and data collection strategy.
- Review schedule of events to confirm full awareness of data capture modalities between EDC and direct from patient data collection.
- Ensure early identification of data collection platforms for EDC, eCOA, and other external data streams.
- Schedule a technology-centric demonstration of all proposed vendors to ensure clarity on their offerings and determine if these meet study requirements.
- Establish standard timelines for contracting with data collection vendors. Failure to establish clarity results in timeline delays.
- Clarity on use of global CRFs – use of global CRFs ensures optimal EDC timelines, in addition to facilitating the Statistics and Programming team efforts.
- Schedule joint KOMs with all vendors and develop a master timeline for the data collection ecosystem (EDC + all vendors where data needs to be integrated into the EDC) to be live to meet FPI visit requirements.
- Provide effective ongoing oversight to all vendors during the ecosystem build. Identify risks and work as a collective team to identify solutions to ensure data collection system goes live as per timelines.
- An ongoing discussion during the EDC build process is whether the build can start from an advanced draft version of the protocol, or if the build should commence when the protocol is fully approved. Starting the build process from an advanced version of the protocol – once the schedule of assessments has been finalized – will allow the team to have valuable time during the build process while the administrative aspects of the protocol are being finalized. This approach should be balanced with the scenario where protocol amendments may be introduced before the protocol is finalized; this situation adds a risk of rework. A cross-functional discussion on the pros and cons of starting the EDC build process from an advanced version of the protocol Vs starting the build from the final version of the protocol should occur as soon as possible.

Data Collection Ecosystem Planning

The Importance of Choosing Fit-For-Purpose Data Collection Tools – A Case Study

A large Clinical Research Organization (CRO) acquired a niche company with a focus on post marketing observational studies. The smaller company had established a strong scientific reputation. Following the acquisition, it

Data collection ecosystem planning

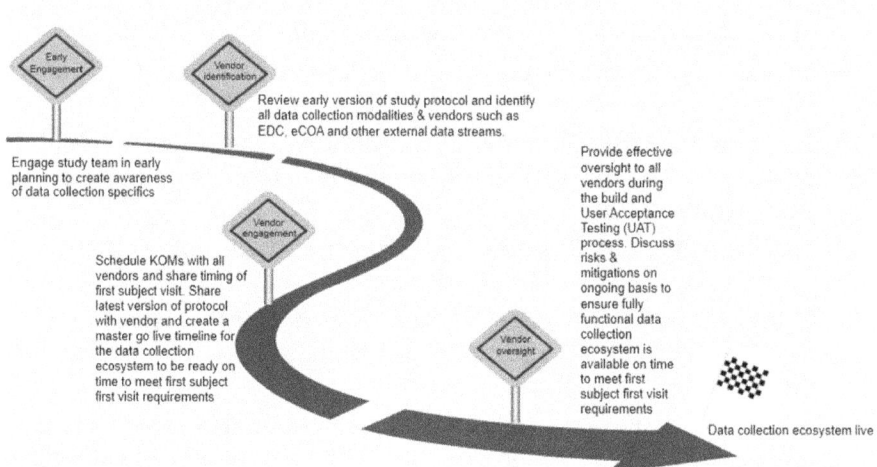

FIGURE 4.3
Data collection ecosystem planning.

was clear that a technology realignment was required. The niche organization had developed an in-house EDC tool that offered significant customizations; the tradeoff was the absence of standard features that are expected from a mainstream EDC tool. This model created challenges during the start-up, conduct, and close-out phases of studies since significant custom programming was required to meet industry expectations. An external consultant was brought in to assess the situation and provide technology recommendations. Following a thorough analysis, the consultant concluded that a modern, flexible platform was important to cater to the unique needs of observational studies. Key considerations that led to this conclusion were as follows:

- Observational studies are non-interventional in design, and ideally data required for the study should be part of standard patient care.
- Patient care is the focus at sites participating in observational studies. Site staff cannot be burdened with cumbersome data collection activities that will impede patient care.
- Data collection solutions on observational studies need to focus on end user experience and ensure intuitive system navigation.
- As increased types of data are being collected via direct-from-subject data collection modalities, the data collection platform should be flexible to integrate external data streams.

Following the assessments, a light EDC platform was successfully deployed for the conduct of observational studies. The solution was received positively by participating sites.

Study Conduct Phase

Challenges: In the quest to get the data collection ecosystem ready prior to first subject visit, the following key requirements may not be fully addressed.

- Metrics reporting – clean patient tracker, missing pages report, audit report
- Protocol amendments – time required to implement protocol amendments ahead of deliverables
- External data transfers – issues with data transfer quality, such as missing variables and data point mapping
- Data integration challenges – issues with external data integration within the EDC
- Data validation algorithms not functioning as per approved data validation specifications, leading to generation of erroneous queries and or needed queries not flagging for certain data anomalies
- Vendor data turnaround times – delays in vendors sending updated versions of data ahead of interim deliverables

Solutions: Study teams should consider the following practices during the early stages of the conduct phase:

- The data flow chart should be included in the Data Management Plan (DMP). The data flow chart will define the data journey visually.
- Obtain missing pages report and clean patient tracker as soon as possible. The reports should be reviewed by the cross-functional study teams to ensure accuracy. Any inconsistencies with these reports should be discussed promptly with the vendor and resolved as a priority.
- Review validation outputs to look for trends that may point to potential issues with programming. Any errors should be discussed promptly with the EDC vendor and resolved as a priority. As a rule, the use of automated validations should be maximized for data review and cleaning, which will reduce dependency on manual listings for data review.
- Obtain clarification and document the decision on the quality checks vendors will perform prior to sending data transfers. Here are a few examples of quality checks that vendors should perform before initiating data transfers. The list is not exhaustive:

- Confirm that the transfer will be sent in accordance with the approved Data Transfer Agreement (DTA)
- Record counts for each transfer
- Ensure all reported issues from the previous transfer have been addressed
- Compare the latest transfer against the previous transfer to confirm that there are no unintended changes in the transfer
- Schedule a planning meeting with all vendors ahead of interim deliverables to discuss expectations on turn-round times to send updated data transfers. This step will ensure there are no delays during interim analysis deliveries.
- Ensure all subject-reported data is reviewed on an ongoing basis by cross-functional team members. This practice will assist in identifying any gaps with subject-reported data. Since subject-reported data cannot be queried, identifying gaps in this data provides an opportunity for the sites to follow up with subjects as needed and ensure better compliance.
- Document data review by cross-functional team members in the study's IDRP. This will ensure that holistic data review is performed as per the frequency defined in the IDRP. Completion of ongoing data review as per the IDRP should be documented clearly.

The Importance of Maintaining Data Currency on Ongoing Basis – A Case Study

During the conduct of a large global study with a lengthy enrollment period, the team discussions around an upcoming interim database lock identified the following issues:

- Large number of open data queries
- Issues with certain data validations not functioning appropriately
- Number of open issues from vendor transfers
- Uncertainty with accuracy of missing pages reports and clean patient reports
- Issues with data transfer format for subject-reported data transfers
- Gaps in subject-reported data

What steps could the study team have taken to avoid this scenario?

- Ongoing review of query ageing reports and follow-up with sites to ensure queries are being addressed on ongoing basis during the study.

- Ongoing review of validation outputs to determine if there are any programming errors.
- Review number of open issues following each vendor data transfer. Follow up with vendors to ensure issues are addressed in subsequent transfers.
- Ongoing review of missing pages reports and clean patient reports to confirm accuracy of reports. Follow up with the vendor in case there are any inconsistencies and ensure prompt resolution.
- Ensure the vendor is providing appropriate metric reports for subject-reported data. Review reports on an ongoing basis to identify trends with missing and or incomplete data. Alert sites with a communication to retrain subjects to ensure they complete data as per protocol mandate.

Study Close-Out Phase

Challenges: Here are some scenarios that may come up very close to a final database lock stage:

- Errors in metric reporting
- Unresolved issues with vendor data transfers
- Issues with sample tracking in instances where one laboratory sends samples to multiple laboratories for analyses
- Inventory challenges with return of tablets issued to subjects for reporting data
- Status of vendor databases after database lock
- Clarifications on database archival at vendor after database lock

Solutions: Following practices are helpful for the teams to plan proactively for on-time, quality database locks:

- Check accuracy of metrics reports on an ongoing basis to avoid last minute surprises with programming errors that may output erroneous metrics.
- Ensure high level of vendor data quality is maintained on ongoing basis. Additionally, vendor data should be integrated into study SDTMs and reviewed on an ongoing basis to confirm vendor data integrity.
- In studies which deploy tablets for data collection, ensure sites retrieve tablets on time and all data has been uploaded into the study database.
- Discuss vendor practices for data archival post database lock to ensure it meets regulatory authorities' requirements.

How Can Study Teams Utilize Technology Effectively to Achieve on-Time, Quality Database Lock?

- Study teams should check the accuracy of metrics reporting on an ongoing basis, especially outputs related to the missing pages reports and clean patient tracker. On studies with multiple external data vendors, clean patient trackers require complex programming, and outputs need to be checked for accuracy.
- Define clear guidelines on how chain of custody will be established when samples are transferred from one laboratory to multiple laboratories for analyses.
- Utilize full capabilities of the supporting technology tools to perform cross-functional, holistic data reviews. These reviews will identify data trends, anomalies, and study-level trends for further investigation.

Supporting Technology Solution Tools

The growing number of data streams in clinical research provides opportunities for holistic review of data. While data validation rules enable review of data at a subject level, presenting the data at a study level to the study teams enables holistic reviews.

Supporting technology solutions offer capabilities to ingest a variety of data from multiple streams and present the combined data in intelligent formats that enable study-level, holistic data review and trend identification. Following are a few examples of study-level data review that can be supported by the supporting technology solutions:

- Overall trend identification at the study level based on pooled data.
- Identify study-level subject safety trends.
- Enable holistic review of selected data points across the entire study at individual subject level, and overall study level.
- Proactive identification of data quality trends.
- In studies that generate subject samples, the supporting technology solution can enable sample tracking flows that allow tracing the sample journey as samples make their way across multiple vendors. The automation avoids the need for multiple teams performing manual sample reconciliations to track chain of custody.
- Complex data reviews that cannot be performed via data validations can be addressed by supporting technology solutions tools, avoiding the need to generate line listings for data review.

The following steps will ensure studies can benefit from the capabilities that the technology solutions tool has to offer:

- List all the standard technology solution offerings in the standard IDRP template. Discuss required solutions for individual studies and alert the technology implementation team about the needs.
- If custom reporting is needed for a study, ensure the expectations are discussed as part of the early engagement process to ensure the solution can be implemented for the study.
- Set a timeline for discussing implementation to ensure the solution is available when the data collection ecosystem goes live.
- Ongoing reviews to check and confirm data ingestion and continuous refreshing of new data from the various data streams are occurring as defined in the study specifications.
- Ensure the technology solution tool implementation team is aware of the date by which the data collection ecosystem needs to be live.
- Study Project Manager needs to check with all cross-functional team members to ensure they are trained in the tool's capabilities.

Summary

Technology plays a pivotal role for CDM. It provides the means to collect data efficiently, review it timely, and analyze it accurately. From a CDM point of view, even without a deep background in information technology, the need to lead the discussion related to the tools required for being able to conduct the study is evident. With the growing landscape of offerings, this might result in a dedicated role, as discussed in Chapter 1, around a CSL, who ensures that data integrity questions and quality by design aspects are being addressed properly.

The expanding role of CDM will become even more evident – and yes, exciting – in the next chapter where we will see the natural evolution from CDM to CDS and the new frontiers we have to conquer.

5

Clinical Data Management Versus Clinical Data Science

With Stephen Cameron

Thus far, we have set the foundation of the importance of CDM and the skill sets which help to ensure the data quality of a clinical trial.

As you know, clinical trials have evolved significantly over the last decade, and with them the discipline of CDM has needed to evolve with it. Further skills ranging from more complex trial designs and a plethora of new technologies to facilitate DCT's as well as Diversity, Equity, and Inclusion (DEI) have resulted in the need for clinical data managers to look at data through a new and more critical lens. Blanketing over all of this, AI and advanced data interrogation methodology are empowering fresh insights and data visualization which were previously considered out of reach.

This expanded skill set has resulted in a new profession branch to emerge: Clinical Data Science. So, what is the difference between CDM and CDS? Let's spend some time together discussing this, focusing on:

- What is CDS and why it isn't CDM?
- Where does clinical trial complexity come into play?
- Is there a demonstrable shift to CDS in our industry?
- Do we still need soft skills?

What Is Clinical Data Science and Why It Isn't Clinical Data Management?

Some may think that CDS is no more than the newest trending title to keep us sounding like we are doing something new instead of the same old data review and quality checks we have been doing for decades. If you have been in the industry as long as I have, you likely have heard many titles describing our clinical data managers. A few examples include Clinical Data Manager,

DOI: 10.1201/9781003648314-5

Lead Data Manager, Clinical Data Lead, Clinical Informatics Manager, Data Program Lead, and CDM Manager. So what makes CDS any different?

When you looked at this group of titles, they were all often doing many of the same core tasks with peripheral roles picking up the full envelope of tasks encompassing CDM. A few examples of additional roles which may be performed by others include data review (CDC), analysis programming (Data Programmer), EDC programming (Clinical System Designer), or budget and forecasting tasks (Project Manager).

If we group these skills together, I like to think of these as the planets within our solar system. As we did in Chapter 2, looking at the atoms of the universe to draw comparisons to our profession, let us look at the sky again – that is, the core skills that make up the foundation of CDM. You can group the planets together to describe the roles you would like within your organization; however, you need the full solar system, including that pesky asteroid belt, to make up the full remit of a Clinical Data Manager and ensure end-to-end integrity of data delivery.

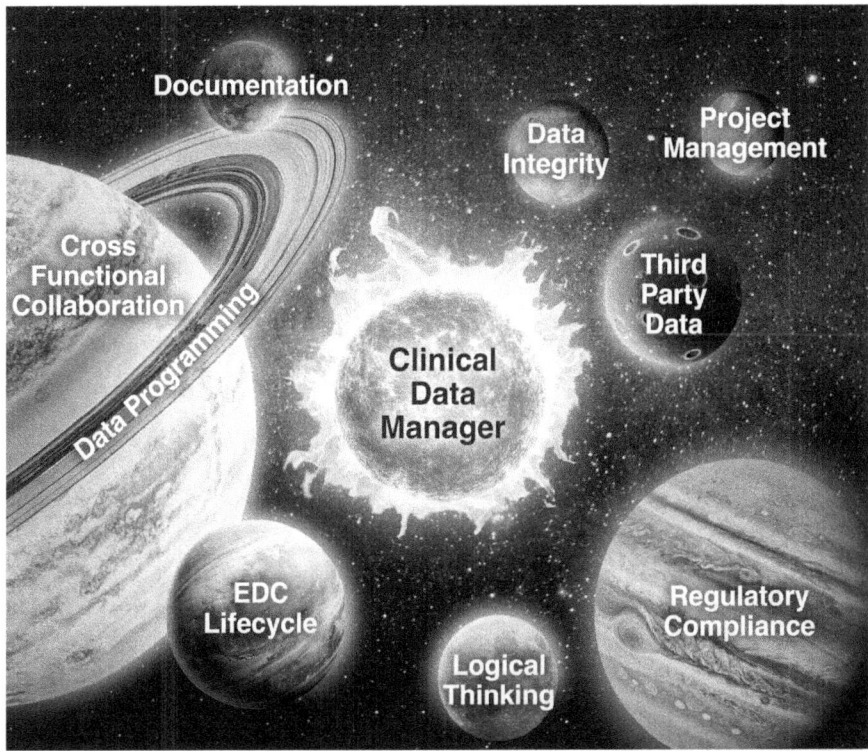

FIGURE 5.1
The CDM sky.

I have chosen the sun in this case to represent the molten core of our Clinical Data Manager, with skills orbiting as celestial bodies around their immense gravitational pull. I know there are many interpretations of these key skills within our industry but for me, those listed are the most significant assets in their skill set. For ease of review, I have also listed them out below.

Skills of a CDM:

- Documentation
- Data integrity
- Third-Party Data
- Data Quality
- EDC Lifecycle
- Data Programming
- Regulatory Compliance
- Logical Thinking
- Cross-functional Collaboration

Why the change from management to science? Clinical Data Managers focus generally on the quality and accuracy of the data. They have strong project management skills and are the masters of the data flow for a clinical trial. They are the gate to data quality and data delivery. There are aspects of critical thinking involved in this role; however, it often has a transactional focus and set framework.

On the other hand, when we think of "science" and the scientific method, we think of the following sequence:

1. Observe
2. Define
3. Hypothesize
4. Test
5. Conclude

After understanding our clinical trial objectives, we are testing our theories (hypothesis) on our outcomes against the evidence we observe through the execution of the clinical trial. We are setting our hypothesis initially through our protocol design and risk assessment. As discussed in the RBQM section, TransCelerate's Risk Assessment and Categorization Tool (RACT) sets this foundation of study risks. It is a useful example here, as it identifies data risks we are going to consider strategies for monitoring and mitigating through the duration of the study. QTLs are another terrific example, where we are setting our data hypothesis and thresholds at the onset of the study. We are looking for the things we don't know yet and exploring them objectively during trial conduct. So what are the skills that are needed to achieve this?

For the skills of a Clinical Data Scientist, we need to not only consider those skills of a Clinical Data Manager but extend our view to the visible stars in our night sky. We can see the same stars in the sky but depending on where we are in the world, we may map and name those constellations differently. In other words, group the skills into different roles and responsibilities within your organizational structure. No matter how we group and name our constellations of skills, we still need all those stars to satisfy the scope of CDS, and those skills are new from those of our foundational CDM. I have simplified this in Figure 5.2. Can you guess what the constellation is spelling and what the symbol is?

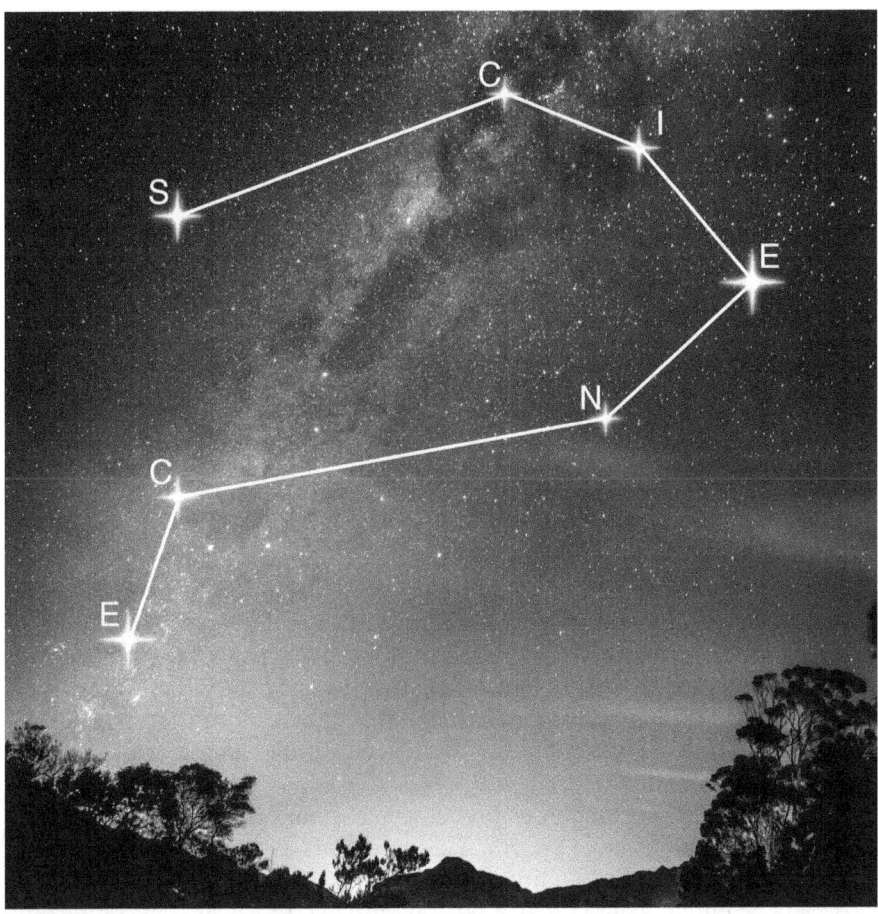

FIGURE 5.2
Symbol in the CDM sky.

Hopefully you spotted that it spelled out "Science". To fill all of the letters of the Clinical Data Scientist skills within the starry night would have been an impressive endeavor with some very small font!

The constellation I chose was a loose interpretation of a question mark. Interestingly, the "?" is not that universal a symbol across languages, as some also use upside down symbols (Spanish), mirrored (Arabic), semi colons (Greek), and an open circle (Armenian) for example. Regardless of which interrogation point is used, they each represent the skillset enhancement welcomed by all critical thinkers. That inquisitive mind of a Clinical Data Scientist, taking in the big picture skyscape representing the vastness of diverse data sources and data points to connect the dots into a meaningful insight which is easily interpreted by their audience. Beyond the critical thinking skill, I have summarized many of the other key skills of a Clinical Data Scientist below.

Skills for CDS:

- CDS
- Risk-Based Clinical Data Management (RBCDM)
- Critical thinking
- Data flow automation
- Data quality
- Decentralized clinical trials (DCTs)
- DEI
- Exploratory analytics
- Trend interpretation and simplification for audience (Trending)
- AI/ML adoption
- ATR
- Advanced protocol deployment

There is a plethora of definitions out there for CDS, but they all orbit around a common theme. CDS brings together clinical data and aggregate analytics to provide meaningful trends and insights into complex trials to empower risk-based informed decisions, data quality, and patient safety. This ultimately leads to meaningful and demonstratable oversight and analysis-ready reliable data for clinical trials. CDS is also different from data science. Let's look at those definitions a bit closer:

Per SCDM, CDS encompasses processes, domain expertise, technologies, data *analytics,* and good CDM practices essential to prompt *decision-making* throughout the life cycle of Clinical Research (SCDM).

A Data Scientist is defined as a person employed to *analyze* and interpret complex digital data, such as the usage statistics of a website, especially in order to assist a business in its *decision-making* (Oxford dictionary).

Both focus on decision-making and analytics; however, CDS shifts from a business focus to emphasizing good CDM practices. They also often will have a higher stringency for accuracy than many data scientists' requirements as patient safety requires greater scrutiny. Data science titles started popping up as function titles in early 2010, but the science title adoption has been much more recent for clinical data professionals. At their core, they both still orbit around data.

As our datasets move to greater and greater sizes as a result of trial complexity, technology sensitivity, and sample frequency, the amount of data points on a clinical trial may seem overwhelming. I find that Mark Watney's quote from Andy Weir's novel, *The Martian*, comes in handy to waylay those initial fears. "In the face of overwhelming odds, I'm left with only one option. I'm gonna have to science the shit out of this". Although we are not typically looking at potato farming in clinical trials, as was the need on the Martian landscape in that novel, we are looking at the vastness of our datasets with a lens based on our scientific hypothesis to focus on the data that matters most. The safety of the patient, the primary and secondary endpoints, the integrity of the data, and the compliance to the protocol.

What does this really mean? How do you look at data based on a hypothesis? Let's look at some examples of each:

- ATR
- Endpoint protection
- QTL
- Protocol compliance

Audit Trail Review Example

Starting first with ATR, a typical ATR would include checking that the right access to EDC was provided for the right individual. This one could likely land in the CDM category. A more analytic-driven example could be to look at the time that access was provided. Perhaps it was the PI who accessed EDC to sign off on their agreement that the data entered meets ALCOA (Attributable, Legible, Contemporaneous, Original and Accurate) expectations. Your hypothesis could be that they are following the GCP regulatory guidelines. The EU guidelines on investigator site monitoring as described in the ICH E6(R3) draft 2.12.5 indicate ". . . The investigator should review and endorse the reported data at milestones agreed upon with the sponsor (e.g., interim analysis)" (https://database.ich.org/sites/default/files/ICH_E6%28R3%29_DraftGuideline_2023_0519.pdf).

If the PI Signature was applied, this could infer that the trial was ready for lock, and everything was good. If you look at the time stamp though, you may find that the PI logged in on the last day of the trial, completed their training to access EDC, and then signed all forms a few minutes later. This raises an eyebrow as to whether they were truly reviewing the data at the end of the trial and whether they were doing so across the trial duration. Regulators are looking at data of this sort and challenging it for good reason. It can't be stated enough times that ATR is not optional; it is a regulatory requirement.

Endpoint Protection Example

Endpoint protection is always a key step in ensuring data integrity and readiness for analysis. A Clinical Data Scientist accomplishes this not only through coordinating the standard reviews described in the edit check plan and integrated data review plan but also through exploratory review and a quality gate review at time of delivery. From a hypothesis perspective, they can assess the key endpoint variables as outlined in the protocol and consider what they would expect that data to look like *before* they review the data. They would be considering what checks are in place already cleaning the data, what the data backlogs may be for entry and review, and what the anticipated "dirtiness" of the data may be. With those thoughts in mind, they would then scour the endpoint data in aggregate to look for anomalies outside of their expected hypothesis of the data – for example, missing disease progression data for an oncology trial.

Expanding further on exploratory review, the Clinical Data Scientist will assess the primary and secondary endpoints as well as safety, efficacy, and dosing parameters of a protocol and cross-check through ad-hoc reports and review whether there are outliers in the data that would not be expected. The review is relatively unstructured by design to allow the Clinical Data Scientist the freedom to not be bound by listings and checks already in place but to instead explore the data to find out whether there are holes or oddities that have passed through the initial nets of classical review and reconciliation. This is also a strong asset when working on studies where a reduced or targeted SDV has been deployed, and on-site monitoring is reduced. Central review can allow earlier insights here as the review is available as soon as entered; however, typically the exploratory review is done on a monthly cadence unless an upcoming delivery warrants more frequent review. So, what can this review reveal?

Some typical outcomes from this review can include issues with data import and integration where a failed integration is not populating in the downstream platform and showing as blank or if a data import is showing missing variables or domains. It can also show where a reviewer may be resolving queries incorrectly and where a divergence from expected data collection is occurring. For example, scheduled visits were moved to unscheduled forms incorrectly or AEs were not queried when reported in duplicate. It can also show emerging trends in the data where outliers are not covered by edit checks or listings and a programmed output is needed to close the gap moving forward for the team. The monthly reviews are important to safeguard the integrity of the data; however, they are not the only time for this review.

It is also recommended that the Clinical Data Scientist perform a high-level review of the data packaged for any sponsor delivery or analysis to cross-check that header data for the outputs. Look for simple aspects like "Is this the right study and sponsor?" and "Is there data in each of the outputs for the columns expected?" Focus once again on the data integrity relating to endpoint data, safety, efficacy, and dosing data is also advised as a risk-based strategy to mitigate down-stream analysis impact keeping in mind that this step is meant as a high-level review only, not a deep dive. Trust me, the time you save by this proactive step is paid back manyfold compared to the documentation and additional steps needed to re-deliver a transfer, rebuild a sponsor, and study team's trust in delivery when things like a blank dataset are posted for delivery or analysis. You can imagine how much further this would be amplified if delivery of incorrect sponsor data occurred. This is much less common for dataset deliveries, although it occurs more frequent than it should when looking at study documentation, so keep an eye out for that as well.

Quality Tolerance Limit Example

As discussed previously, QTLs are a key asset for a clinical trial to monitor key analytes during a clinical trial proactively. QTLs are used to monitor subject safety and/or the reliability of trial outcomes; this is a regulatory requirement. They should monitor CTQ factors which jeopardize patient wellbeing and/or the reliability and interpretability of the study. It is key that they are established before FPI. This provides the clinical team with the ability to establish an unbiased hypothesis of what thresholds should be set to. Implementation of QTLs should be described by the sponsor and important breaches reported in the CSR, including actions taken. Clearly, there is not a single stakeholder defining a QTL, but instead, meant to be a cross-functional discussion of which QTLs should be implemented for the study. The approach must include statistical, medical, and cross-functional assessments based on the unique needs of the specific study and is typically grouped into three categories per ICH E6 R2:

- Subject safety
- Systematic issue(s)
- Reliability of the trial

https://database.ich.org/sites/default/files/E6_R2_Addendum.pdf page 21

For example, the expectancy of Serious Adverse Events (SAEs) for an oncology study would be different than that of a pain medication study. Taking an oncology study for example, a potential QTL could be around SAE frequency. Setting an expected threshold (the hypothesis) for the number of SAEs for the study at baseline will allow early warning of a potential/projected QTL breach. This is accomplished through not only reporting actual occurrences cumulatively on a monthly basis and comparing them to the original assumed SAE rate for the study, but also forecasting out what the future trend is, including high and low error bars based on current trending data. This allows time to impact the forecasted trend potentially prior to the QTL breach by reviewing the cause of the current trend and to implement corrective action where possible to bend the curve before the breach occurs. Key to this is to have the clinical data scientist bring these early warning insights to the cross-functional team in a meaningful and clearly understood graph or output so trending can be easily communicated cross-functionally. Understanding why the study may be trending above or below the projected trend can be further explored by looking at the types of SAEs and whether there may be adjustments to the protocol/dosing, education, or visit parameters to enhance safety on the trial or if trial discontinuation may be on the horizon due to emerging safety risks.

Protocol Compliance Example

As we shift to risk-based central monitoring, on-site monitoring is refined and reduced. Two commonly included on-site monitoring strategies are targeted and reduced SDV. Targeted SDV looks at particular data points across a subject for all subjects. This normally targets safety, dosing, and endpoint data deemed most critical for analysis by the biostatistician, sponsor, and cross-functional team. Reduced SDV looks at 100% of all subject data for a designated ratio of subjects at each site. The ratio is once again determined by the biostatistician, sponsor, and cross-functional team and could be 1 in 3 subjects (the first is always 100% SDVed) for a complex indication like an oncology trial or 1 in 5 subjects for a simpler indication, like perhaps a pain relief trial.

Targeted SDV has been utilized for many years now but runs the risk in monitoring that you are missing the notes on a seemingly unrelated source document which could contain relevant data for that critical variable. For example, a patient could note they didn't come to a visit due to a miscarriage, but this was not collected as an entry on the AE form. A miscarriage could be an AE of special interest (AESI) with potential clinical significance or impact on patient safety and the safety profile of the drug.

Reduced SDV should catch this if the subject was in the sample SDVed as all source documentation is verified for the selected subjects and the first subject is always monitored as a minimum. The ratio of patients monitored on site can be adjusted at the subject or trial level (more or less subjects) based on ongoing risk review meetings. Whether you choose 100%, Reduced or Targeted SDV, all should have a risk assessment at the beginning of the trial and establish as your working hypothesis which strategy is your best-fit SDV strategy for your clinical trial.

Why am I giving you all of this background on monitoring strategies? What does it have to do with CDM and CDS? These strategies are risk-based, and the intent is to reduce the risk and not to add risk. The empowerment of analytics and CDS is this role leverages centralized analytics to assess outliers and communicate those trends.

Let's look at a specific example around protocol deviations. The hypothesis was that the reporting of protocol deviations and important protocol deviations should be the same frequency for subjects monitored centrally or on site. During regular risk review meetings, it was found in most studies within a portfolio that the ratios were quite similar for protocol deviations, with deviations reported typically at least slightly higher when monitored on site. A handful of studies had a wider margin, as much as a five-fold difference, when looking specifically at SDV versus central monitoring.

What was the cause of this difference? Is this a case to abandon central monitoring? Surely protocol deviations are key to be reported for a study and should be consistent regardless of the monitoring strategy deployed. When the team investigated, there were many factors at play which had varying degrees of significance. This portfolio involved a blended team where the CRO provided clinical and analytics support and data services were performed by the sponsor. It was found that for the best-reporting studies the sponsor was communicating important protocol deviations (PDs) to the clinical team for follow-up and entry as applicable into the PD database. Listings were also provided to the clinical team to reconcile deviations. For those studies with greater disparity, it was found that a clear reporting mechanism between DM and clinical was not in place so it relied on central review and the monitoring of subjects independently. There was no preamble designator in the query text to flag to the review team that there was a query related to a possible protocol deviation. When anomalies were being flagged through the analytics reviews, including exploratory reviews on endpoints, dosing, and safety data, the team was not keeping up with the entered backlog for follow-up and the deviation process through entry for those flagged took additional time compared to PD's identified during on-site SDV visits. This appeared to further amplify the apparent variance between the reporting frequency. Once the team understood the cause for these differences, trends improved on the portfolio.

So, in summary, it is encouraged that a preamble text similar to "possible protocol deviation" is included in the DM query text in EDC to help differentiate deviation queries for follow-up with the clinical and medical teams. It is key that the departments do not work in isolation but collaborate during risk review meetings to strategize on the best action to take for follow-up when a deviation trend has been identified. This may include site education, changing the monitoring frequency, addition of edit checks, and enhancement of communication pathways around PDs and IPDs. Lastly, a key risk indicator (KRI) around PD and IPD reporting for studies utilizing a reduced SDV monitoring strategy is recommended to be added to your analytics outputs if you are deploying a reduced SDV methodology.

We've talked a bit about the role of the clinical data manager and the evolution of risk-based methodologies they support. Another key evolution which continues to launch across our trials is the evolving design of the trials themselves. Let's take a look at what advanced trials look like today and how a Clinical Data Scientist adds value to these new formats of clinical trials.

Where Does Clinical Trial Complexity Come Into Play?

Thankfully, we have come a long way from the days of paper-based trials, although there remain some holdouts in our data collection journey where paper records still exist. These are typically narrowed to PROs or as a transitory record for home health visits. Knowing where these aspects may come into play and that there may be a potential source data entry error in places we may historically have not considered is only one of the factors to look at for clinical trial design as you map out your data flow diagram for your trial.

As we have moved further into the realm of electronic data in clinical trials, the types of data sources, amount of data collected, and the versatility of trial designs continue to evolve. They can cover multiple indications under one investigational drug (basket), multiple drugs for one indication (umbrella), decentralized and multi-modal trials to enhance DEI, as well as the ability to pivot with mid-stream amendments to increase likelihood of a successful outcome. This has allowed for greater flexibility in trial deployment but has also tended to further burden the sites and subjects with a bolus of new technologies to deal and to comply with. Our regulators continue to provide updated guidance to frame trial options with the intent of enough leeway to allow for innovation without jeopardizing the safety of the patient or integrity of the clinical trial. Before we talk more about what a clinical data scientist can do about all of this amazing data, let's go into greater detail around these types of trials, which are currently grouped into the category of Master Protocol by the National Institute of Health (Glossary – Toolkit (nih.gov)). For ease of reference, I have included each key definition below.

Master Protocol

A master protocol is a trial design that tests multiple drugs and/or multiple subpopulations in parallel under a single protocol, without the need to develop new protocols for every trial. The term "master protocol" is often used to describe the design of such trials, with terms such as "umbrella", "basket", or "platform" describing specific designs.

(Master protocol – Toolkit [nih.gov])

Umbrella Protocol

An umbrella protocol refers to a type of master protocol designed to evaluate multiple investigational therapies administered as single drugs or as drug combinations in a single disease population. Umbrella trials can employ randomized controlled designs to compare the activity of the therapy being studied with a common control arm. The therapy chosen as the control arm for the randomized substudy or substudies should be the standard of care (SOC) for the target population. Thus, the control arm may change over time if newer therapies replace the SOC.

(Umbrella protocol – Toolkit [nih.gov])

Basket Protocol

A basket protocol is a type of master protocol designed to test a single investigational therapy or therapy combination in patients from different disease groups or subgroups in the same clinical trial. The populations in the different "baskets" may be defined by disease, disease stage, histology, number of prior therapies, genetic variants, other biomarkers, or demographic characteristics (such as age). Basket trials may allow new drugs to be tested and approved more quickly than traditional clinical trials.

(Basket protocol – Toolkit [nih.gov])

Platform Protocol

A platform protocol refers to a type of master protocol that tests multiple, targeted therapies for a single disease simultaneously. Platform protocols often include an adaptive design that may eliminate or add treatments based on interim analysis.

(NCImetathesaurus)

Adaptive Design

Protocols can also be set up to allow for adaptive design.

Adaptive design gives a clinical trial to adjust its design in response to information gained throughout the clinical trial. In adaptive design, patient outcomes are measured and analyzed at specific points throughout the trial. Changes to the study design may be implemented based on these observations. Types of modifications include targeting a specific subpopulation of patients, ending a trial early, adjusting sample size, reducing the number of trial arms, changing study endpoints, and modifying dose and/or treatment duration. Adaptive design may provide a more ethical, efficient, and informative alternative to traditional, fixed-design, randomized controlled trials.

(Adaptive design – Toolkit [nih.gov])

Knowing each type of protocol and complex design will help your understanding in the scope of the clinical trial(s) you are running and where potential cross-portfolio risks may emerge. This adds another layer to the aggregated data review complexity as the sponsor may be looking at multiple investigational products added mid-study or across multiple studies on their portfolio. Depending on their teams, they may have more than one Clinical Research Organization supporting their portfolio or aspects of their portfolio – for example, shared clinical site monitoring by more than one CRO. As a Clinical Data Scientist, it is key that you are able to bring all appropriate stakeholders to the table to discuss emerging data trends and insights as well as sharing solutions when cross-portfolio trending may be needed. This is exactly what was occurring for the protocol deviation example mentioned earlier where we expanded our investigation across other trials in the same indication as one of our assessment strategies. What about upcoming deliveries?

When considering the trials being run by a sponsor, one of the key deliveries to think about planning for is the annual DSUR (Development Safety Update report), which is a common standard for periodic annual reporting on drugs under development among ICH regions. It should provide safety information from all ongoing clinical trials and other studies that the sponsor is conducting or has completed during the review period (https://www.ema.europa.eu/en/documents/scientific-guideline/ich-guideline-e2f-development-safety-update-report-step-5_en.pdf). Coordinating the delivery timing of data to align with this DSUR delivery will be a key annual milestone which can extend across multiple studies and, if your team is co-mingled across those studies, will need to be planned for well in advance so that appropriate resourcing and coordination can occur.

As your trials evolve through protocol amendments, you will want to pause to perform a thorough review of the impact any amendment has on your CRF, edit checks, listings, and third-party data review as well as looping in your functional team leads to weigh in on any impacts to their areas. Stats can be significantly impacted in their down-stream programming and analysis. This is similar to what a Clinical Data Manager would be doing historically, but is nonetheless an important step to take. For these complex protocol designs, you will also want to think about updates you made to your data collection and data flow diagram which may be relevant across other arms under the overarching master protocol and also share within the protocol any lessons learned so that the team is able to continue to grow in experience. When looking at types of master protocols, key points of focus should be around the visit structure and dynamic population as well as functionality of study arms for each technology utilized function appropriately. Drop down lists allowing selection of all indication-specific visits and results are also key areas of complexity you should be mindful of in your trial design deployment oversight.

Although a bit of a stretch beyond the typical stakeholder team for trial design and closeout, taking opportunities to invite site staff and more importantly, the patient to offer perspectives on what they believe represents trial participation success and if there were any form design considerations to make the patient or site staff experience better can also have a significant return for the sponsor. As a particularly poignant example, at the SCDM 2024's annual leadership forum, Dr Marilyn Neault, PhD, shared her insights on CRF design for a clinical trial on Parkinson's disease. Key insights shared that resounded with me were on the influence of age in participation and on CRF design and visit frequency. For age, she indicated that at an earlier age, she was more willing to take additional steps that would impact to her daily routine when it came to trying new drugs as there could be potential drug-drug interactions which would take significant time to stabilize or reset should they be considered intolerable. Later in life, this became a more-significant ask as her routine was a known and more-predictable entity so the potential impact to the routine needed a significant return on investment to participate. The second example around CRF design related to a form where she was being asked to complete a form with very small fields. As a Parkinson's patient with frequent tremors, she needed to use a ruler to help guide her hand to complete the form and a form considering the common symptoms of her disease could have been designed for greater ease of completion. Compounding this was the requirement to complete this task every half hour.

So, what's the takeaway? Go beyond the assumption that the data collection strategy for your study is set in stone and reach out to the end users for their insight. You may not always be able to accommodate but sharing with them the "why" can also help with adoption and compliance in that entry. This also is a terrific gateway to the wider topic of DCTs, where there are more options to bring clinical trials to the patient to reduce their burden. Don't worry, we'll dive into that topic in the next chapter! Before we do, we've spent a while hypothesizing that the new role of CDS is the next role evolution in our industry, but where is the proof of this hypothesis? Let's investigate further.

Is There a Demonstratable Shift to CDS in Our Industry?

Now that we understand some of the differentiators between a CDM and a CDS, let's dig into the specific skill sets a bit further. SCDM has summarized this within their paper on "The Evolution of Clinical Data Management into Clinical Data Science" (2020_Evolution-of-CDM-to-CDS-Part-3-Evolution-of-CDM-Role.pdf [scdm.org]). I have paraphrased the key skills in Table 5.1, noting that they are further compressed into common categories compared to my earlier list of skills when introducing each role in this chapter:

SCDM's competency framework is also a useful guide (ref. CDS 101):

TABLE 5.1

Key Skills of a Clinical Data Manager and Clinical Data Scientist

Clinical Data Manager	Clinical Data Scientist
Logic-focused strategic thinking	Analytic and risk-based critical thinking
Transactional data review	Aggregate and exploratory data review
Focus on data integrity	Focus on data quality
Often paired with 100% SDV	Targeted or reduced SDV paired with central SDV
Technology fairly stable	Technology advancing quickly (AI/ML)

Looking at these skills, there is a fundamental shift in the way we look at the data from a data accuracy and integrity focus to a holistic data quality mindset. There are numerous technological advances which are automating every link in the chain from proposal through to Clinical Study Report. With those automations, you would anticipate the need for straightforward steps reduced from a manual human process to a human-in-the-loop automated implementation which requires less time and effort by humans.

There are many examples of this already occurring. One of my favorites is triangular review, where we look at AEs, Concomitant Medications (ConMeds), and Medical History (MedHis) to verify their linkage. For example, if a medication was indicated as being taken for an AE, was the AE present? This is key for the safety of the investigational product but historically a very cumbersome process as you would need to have the AE, ConMeds, and MedHis pages open on your screens and flipping between them to match up dates and potential overlaps. It is also challenging for sites to resolve these queries as they are, by nature, crossing multiple forms within EDC. The automation of this process to suggest potential queries for the data reviewer has the potential to save significant time and also reduce the risk of human error by refining the number of review items to those per the data that appear truly variant. Auto-coding further enhances this process by reducing the manual coding effort to a handful of terms that were not able to auto-code. As these systems continue to evolve with the refinement support of human review, time will continue to compress. This also ultimately leads to fewer erroneous queries to the sites and enhanced patient safety as queries will be sent faster to the sites for resolution.

Another area of emphasis for vendors to search for solutions is the direct ingestion of the protocol to auto-generate a CRF and EDC build recommendations with CDISC standardization to enhance efficiency in analysis and regulatory delivery. This allows the database build team to focus on design and deployment of the more nuanced forms of the study. There are also numerous vendors championing central data repositories to connect EDC data with an ever-growing list of third-party data (wearable devices, ePRO, Central Labs, specialty labs, etc.) and other data sources like CDMS, eTMF, resourcing, and finance applications. This intuits the shift from CDM to CDS to expand to support stakeholders and other data users as well. The clinical research space is risk-averse and thus historically slow to adapt to changes. Currently, only around half of sponsors adopt a monitoring strategy other than 100% SDV for their trials. So, where's the proof to substantiate the hypothesis that the shift is occurring?

At the 2023 SCDM annual conference in San Diego, Brian McCourt, from Duke Clinical Research Institute (DCRI), shared a trend analysis of this question, sampling organizational trending data for the number of positions in junior and senior roles within historical CDM roles as well as CDS and clinical informatics roles. His organization made a conscious pivot in 2019 and reflected a consistent growth in new roles in CDS, although at a lower overall number. In comparison, legacy CDM roles remain needed but are continuing to decline in prevalence, with the majority now being senior staff. In 2022, there was an inflection point and now there are more CDS's than CDM's in his organization. He noted that this was a long and slow transition to adjust with the speed of the portfolio change but has been accelerating along with the adoption of new data sources, tools, and methodologies.

Speaking to other organizations, this shift in roles to weigh toward the Clinical Data Scientist from the Clinical Data Manager is not isolated. This is further amplified regionally where high-cost regions still require the leadership-skilled CDS roles, but the feeding junior roles are shifted to mid- or low-cost regions. This has created a growing gap in North America, for example, for new hires to come in at the CDS level as they will not have prior experience in the field when they graduate. Immigration from low- and mid-cost regions as well as remote working global solutions help somewhat; however, a more permanent country-specific solution is needed to guide our next generation of Clinical Data Scientists.

Options like associate levels are one such avenue, where the critical analytic mindset can be enhanced through specialized onboarding and job-shadowing with seasoned CDS. Even more encouraging is the expanding reference library for continuing learning within the CDS space (ACDM, SCDM, JSCDM), as well as emerging educational programs specific to CDS. One example in development by Professor Richard Ittenbach is the Master of Science in CDS program he is developing. Details of the proposed curriculum are showcased in Figure 5.3.

He notes in his paper that 85% of the workforce currently have bachelor's degrees, with 5% holding a 2-year diploma as there are no formal requirements to enter the profession. With the specialized needs of the evolving role, the unmet demand in high-cost regions is felt in the recruiting pipeline. Providing a more advanced degree to facilitate stepping directly into the CDS role would be a tremendous asset to our industry. We have rightly established a seat at the table with the hands-on growth of our skill sets; however, we are often mismatched in qualifications when looking at our medical and statistical counterparts at the table. Bringing advanced degrees

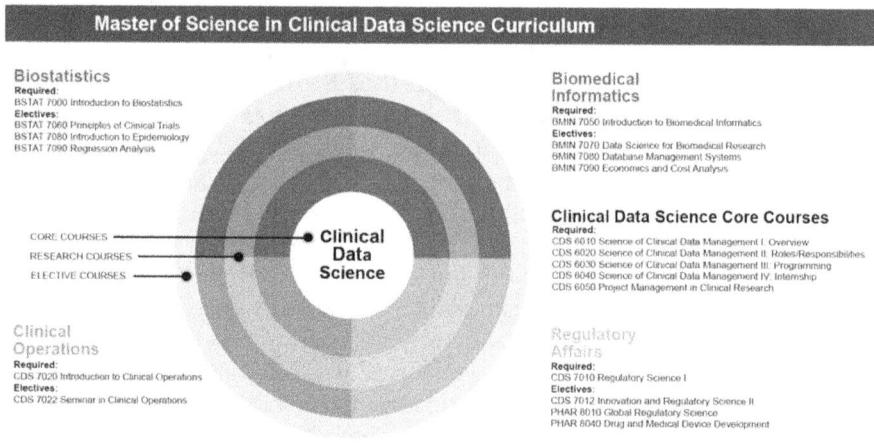

FIGURE 5.3

Ittenbach RF. From clinical data management to clinical data science. Clin Trans Sci. 2023; 16(8): 134–135.

Image modified to greyscale with permission of author.

forward would help to further balance the legs of the advanced table we collaborate at.

Clearly, bolstering our knowledge in the core disciplines of biostats and clinical operations will serve us well in communicating with those stakeholders and augment our ability to think critically and strategically about the data journey and data quality. Biomedical informatics and regulatory affairs are lockstep with the core of CDS skills and together represent a well-rounded CDS toolset that employers would find as assets for new hires to hold knowledge of. So, what of the soft skills we think of that are associated with the CDM role? Are they being lost as we shoulder the burden of our technical prowess?

Do We Still Need Soft Skills?

When we think of soft skill requirements of a CDS, not only are they present, they are becoming even more vital as well. Professor Ittenbach's proposed syllabus highlights that critical thinking resonates as a fundamental thread and competency. Soft skills also resound as a vital aspect of a Clinical Data Scientist. Let's have a look at what those soft skills could look like for some of the role's specific areas of focus:

TABLE 5.2

Comparison of Clinical Data Scientist Areas of Focus and Soft Skills

Clinical Data Scientist Area of Focus	Soft Skills
Analytic and risk-based critical thinking	Communication and collaboration, leadership, critical thinking
Aggregate and exploratory data review	Observation, communication, adaptability, creativity, critical thinking
Focus on data quality	Communication and collaboration, integrity
Central data review augmenting Source Data Verification	Communication and collaboration, critical thinking
Technology advancement (AI/ML)	Communication and collaboration, adaptability, empathy
Complex trial deployment	Communication and collaboration, adaptability

As you can see from Table 5.2, communication and collaboration are the unifying theme and a core vital asset for any clinical data manager. Let's work through each of these categories of soft skills in greater detail with specific examples.

- Critical Thinking
- Communication and Collaboration
- Leadership
- Social Skills (adaptability, empathy, integrity)

Critical Thinking

Critical thinking is where the science of CDS comes into full shine. Although this skill is not unique to CDS, and according to the foundation for critical thinking has been around for 2,500 years, the what and how are unique when it comes to the clinical trial framework. Let's take the bulleted summary as outlined by Richard Paul and Linda Elder in 2008:

A Well-Cultivated Critical Thinker

- raises vital questions and problems, formulating them clearly and precisely;
- gathers and assesses relevant information, using abstract ideas to interpret it effectively;
- comes to well-reasoned conclusions and solutions, testing them against relevant criteria and standards;

- thinks open-mindedly within alternative systems of thought, recognizing and assessing, as need be, their assumptions, implications, and practical consequences; and

- communicates effectively with others in figuring out solutions to complex problems.

> Critical thinking is, in short, self-directed, self-disciplined, self-monitored, and self-corrective thinking. It presupposes assent to rigorous standards of excellence and mindful command of their use. It entails effective communication and problem solving abilities and a commitment to overcome our native egocentrism and sociocentrism.
>
> (Richard Paul and Linda Elder, *The Miniature Guide to Critical Thinking Concepts and Tools*, Foundation for Critical Thinking Press, 2008)

In other words, critical thinking is a cyclical lifecycle where you start with identifying the question/problem statement, reason through the supporting data/information associated with the problem and decide on how you can evaluate your hypothesis. You then test your hypothesis and analyze the outcome, whereupon you restart the cycle if further questions surface to allow for further refinement. Figure 5.4 is a good example of this cycle.

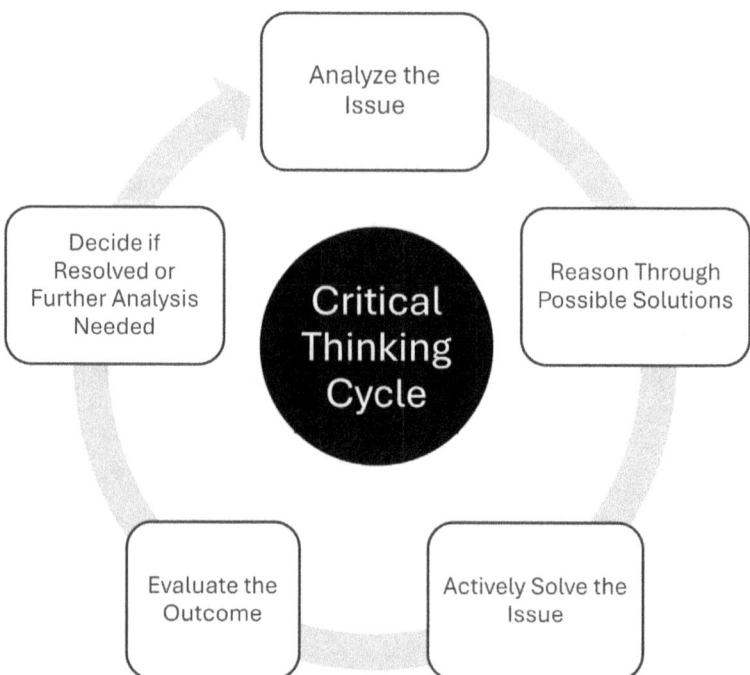

FIGURE 5.4
Critical Thinking Cycle.

This is not only an individual cycle but also a cross-functional experience for clinical trials, where you have to complete the cycle and convey your outcomes to your stakeholders in a consumable format so they can collaborate on next steps for mitigation or resolution of the issue at hand. Let's talk some more about communication.

Communication and Collaboration

Communication and collaboration are not only the need to articulate your thoughts on the data trends you are surfacing through RBQM but also to do so through collaboration with cross-functional stakeholders to gather the combined data assets into a format which will be consumable by the intended audience. This can vary drastically from one stakeholder to the next. For example, if a wearable device dataflow is disrupted, bringing the technical team together to outline specifically where the issue is being observed in detailed technical terms will be of utmost value. Documentation here is key so teams are very clear on steps through resolution. You need to simplify that aspect to an overall summary when bringing updates to the wider cross-functional team and further refining if the issue has a financial or delivery risk and an escalation to the executive is needed. In the latter case, I recommend breaking down to a few groupings: Issue, Root Cause, Impact, and Mitigation. This is a similar format a CDM would utilize.

Where communication skills diverge would be at risk review meetings. In this setting, you are often the center stage for CDS risk and issue management. Your analytics and exploratory reviews can be very in depth as you explore the evolving data in aggregate against protocol expectations, KRIs and QTLs. Simply stating that the blood pressure for a subject is an outlier from other subjects is not sufficient. Visually representing that through a scatter plot diagram can help translate that knowledge to the cross-functional team. Layering on further details around the visit and other factors surrounding concomitant medications, dose administration, and other AEs can help paint the full picture for clinical and medical team's collaborative assessment of actions to take. This all takes professionalism and storytelling to deliver your communications effectively. Take a leadership stance that welcomes collaboration and cement your chair at the table as a meaningful contributor. In so doing, you will be able to deliver your messaging effectively.

Leadership

Leadership is multi-fold for a Clinical Data Scientist. Often time you need to pivot your leadership style to the situation at hand. This is a common skill with the Clinical Data Manager in many ways as we look at team interactions and delivery laterally to other functional team leads and vertically to both your CDS team and your executive leadership. Where it differs, I think, are the topics of Risk-Based Quality Data Management, data trending, automation, and visualization, which has accelerated in the field of CDS over the last half decade or so for clinical trials. A part of this will land in the social skills to be discussed shortly, but from a leadership perspective, it is important to have a visible presence as early as possible in the clinical trial development cycle. This can be at the protocol design phase or the RFP. In doing so, you allow yourself the opportunity to share timely and impactful insights on data flow, indication-specific considerations, data standards, risk and mitigation strategies relating to data management, reporting, visualization, and data currency options that will best-fit the study design. If you are not actively engaging, as a leader, your important voice will be lost at the table.

Leadership doesn't mean who has the loudest voice. Instead, think about what assets you can bring to the audience you are engaging with and what format of communication will best suit each situation. If you are engaging with your executive audience, bullet it to succinct discussion points along with risks, mitigations, and timeline impacts. If you are collaborating with functional team leads, consider their background expertise and the specific value they will get out of your information. Tailor the storytelling of your interaction to align with their needs and key engagement points so that the conversation remains relevant. Listen as well. Remember that you are not the expert in all fields and they will have welcomed insights to share if they are brought into the conversation to share their perspective. This is one of the most vital parts of risk-based CDM as that cross-functional lens allows a best-fit plan to be applied to each emerging risk or study consideration. There will be times when getting that engagement will be hard-fought until the value of the interaction is fully understood. Thinking of leadership, I often think back to how the military works through critical engagements when time is of the essence. This parallels with clinical trials in many ways, as timelines are often paramount to achieving analysis milestones and optimizing the analysis and registrational lifecycle of a clinical trial in a highly competitive landscape.

An excellent leadership strategy which I have deployed countless times is that your initial plan doesn't need to be perfect when you encounter a roadblock to your delivery. Consider the quick and known wins you can deploy your team to address while you outline the detailed plan for the issue at hand. Say, for example, a new analyte is added to a mid-stream study which requires retrospective entry and upon migration, fires thousands of discrepancies. Assuming you had planned for this but perhaps underestimated the full impact of the fallout and have a looming delivery. Initially, your heart may sink as you envision the effort needed to resolve the missing fields of data by your data management team. You know there are many unrelated queries that also need to be resolved by the team so you can guide them to those immediate tasks while you consider alternative strategies with the clinical and project management team. In doing so, you have allowed the team to work in parallel while you work out the more detailed plan. Perhaps the clinical team resolves the entries directly with the sites and queries are closed by the system. Perhaps you add a delay of a week or two for sites to enter the data after they are provided updated CRF Completion Guidelines and a site newsletter spotlighting the entry needs. If timelines are compressed, perhaps you need to expand your team to accommodate the bolus. Remember firstly that you are never alone on a clinical trial. You have not only your study stakeholders but also your management team, peers, and executive leadership should the need be warranted. Seeking support and consultation is not a sign of weakness in my mind; it is an opportunity to extend and achieve. In order to reach out to these assets in your network, you will also need to have strong social skills.

Social Skills

We all are unique in our personal view of our social skills. Whether we are introverts or extroverts, we need to adapt to and adopt our audience, be it individual, team, leadership, or an external professional interaction. As a Clinical Data Scientist, you likely will be placed into each of these settings. As a result of the Clinical Data Scientist role taking on these new skills and responsibilities, I have found that the need to advocate across study stakeholders and within your own organization the merits and regulatory importance of Risk-Based CDM can have a positive impact toward adoption and the teams' effective cross-functional interactions to achieve quality data in delivery.

Being an advocate for this adoption will likely need to continue for the next half century while further traction is attained. Looking at Steve Young's article in Applied Clinical Trials (*October 15, 2024, Applied Clinical Trials-10-01-24 Volume 33, issue 10*), he highlights that adoption has risen from 47% to 77% per Association of Clinical Research Organizations (ACRO) at the end of 2020, but Tufts Center for the Study of Drug Development, in collaboration with CluePoints and PWC found that adoption of RBQM, was only 57% in 2023. Larger organizations were found to have higher adoption (63%) compared to those running 25–100 clinical trials (59%). Working in a Clinical Research Organization, I have seen similar trending and have had lengthy discussions.

In one particular instance, a sponsor slowly shifted their mindset to adoption of a risk-based mentality and methodology over a 3-year span. Initially, they considered 100% Source Data Verification their risk strategy and were slow to adopt regulatory guidance around the establishment of QTLs and other central review strategies when they adjusted below the 100% SDV threshold. After a three-year journey they not only have embraced the RACT tool and deployed QTLs but also established an internal department and analytics solution in support of Risk-Based Quality Management. Likely you will also get tapped to speak to AI and ML, and what human-in-the-loop means while everyone works to adopt aspects of these emerging data and technology tools. More on that will be shared in the coming chapters.

For now, your social skills to engage your teams, stakeholders, and leadership contacts can be further enhanced by considering that the media of communication can also be multi-modal. You may find some team members enjoy an analog email communication to assist with potential language barriers while others may want a phone call or video call so that tone and expressions can be interpreted. I also encourage you to expand your horizon beyond your local team and engage in a volunteer society like CDISC, ACDM, SCDM, TransCelerate, or any of the professional organizations within our profession so you can hear the opinions and experiences of other thought leaders as well as embrace opportunities to share your knowledge with your peers and next generation of Clinical Data Scientists. It may be out of your comfort zone to start, but trust me, it is well worth it!

Summary

Thank you for jumping on the light ship to the stars and this huge leap forward from the Clinical Data Manager to the Clinical Data Scientist. We looked at the intricacies of both roles, the key differentiators, and foundational "why" of the need for the role evolution. We substantiated the hypothesis that the role of Clinical Data Scientist is indeed taking traction in our industry and that there is evolving training available to support and facilitate its growth. Lastly, we considered the continuing relevance of the importance of soft skills for the role and what socialization aspects of our evolving clinical trial space hold the greatest relevance for you as the voice of the Clinical Data Scientist.

We will now shift to the topic of Decentralized Clinical Trials. Other names for these types of trials have circulated over the last decade like Virtual and Digitized Clinical Trials, but there is a reason why "Decentralized" has stuck. Join me in the next chapter to find out why this is the most significant trial evolution of all time and how it directly addresses DEI within clinical trials.

6

Demystifying DCTs (Decentralized Clinical Trials)

With Emily Mitchell

Here, we will review exactly what a DCT is as defined by regulatory authorities and the mindset shift CDMs need to embrace for success. We will review whether DCTs are the next best thing, since sliced bread, or if the allure is wearing off as society turns back to normal post-pandemic. Some of this will be further explored with a positive pre-pandemic case study and one not so successful post-pandemic study. We'll look at what went wrong and how it could have been prevented.

The goal for us is to understand the change CDMs need to make in approaching decentralized data and the cautionary elements that should not be forgotten.

As we think about the future, we will also touch on what decentralizing data has the potential to become and implications to clinical trials and medicine as a result.

In this chapter, we will cover the following topics:

- DCTs – how we got here and the future
- Whether DCTs are really the way of the future
- The changes for CDMs with DCTs

DCTs – How We Got Here, Now What?

One of the most important first steps in accepting DCTs is understanding exactly what a DCT is and how broad of a definition it encompasses. The FDA has released a guidance document for conducting clinical trials with decentralized elements. The FDA defines "decentralized elements can include, among other things, telehealth visits with trial personnel, in-home visits with remote trial personnel, or visits with local health care providers". They define DCTs as "a clinical trial that includes decentralized elements

DOI: 10.1201/9781003648314-6

where trial-related activities occur at locations other than traditional clinical trial sites" (Conducting Clinical Trials With Decentralized Elements | FDA).

Now that we have laid out what the definition of a decentralized element is and the overarching DCT, what does that mean and how did we get here? Many think that the idea of decentralized trials started when the COVID-19 pandemic hit the world and stay-in-place orders were mandated. In actuality, the first decentralization of a clinical trial was conducted by Pfizer in 2011, but the foundations had been laid in 2007.

While this Pfizer trial was less than ideal:

- Screening process through the internet
- Participants managing their own trial activity
- Participants reporting clinical data results directly to the trial investigator (vs. the physician measuring them, i.e., temperature, weight, height)

It did lead to many valuable teachings. This was the first attempt to validate the patient-centered approach in clinical research.

The point of data capture has started to move closer to the patient. As CDM there are some parts of the above approach that frankly scare me. Where is the oversight? Are the assessments being conducted consistently? Who can review the data? How do they review the data? Is it considered validated data? We'll explore thoughts on these questions a bit later.

Let's go back to 2020 and to the infamous COVID-19 pandemic. The world essentially shut down in March of 2020, to the likes of which no one in modern medicine had seen. What did this mean for trial participants and their visits? How was the care of patients going to continue without further spreading this deadly virus? Is there such a thing as a global protocol deviation? Quickly companies pivoted and became creative with solutions to still oversee patients' safety, that is, the primary purpose of medical care after all. Telehealth visits were scheduled, and patients were seen, but there was a larger underlying issue.

What about the protocol required assessments? How could we conduct a laboratory draw remotely, what if additional drug was needed, what if drug could only be administered by the physician? Now is where creativity came into play with hospital pharmacy staff turning into curriers, the adoption of home health nursing skyrocketed (and so did the cost), and looking at ways to remotely monitor data like vital signs via wearables and sensors.

All are valid points and very important questions to answer; however, there is the fundamental data question. How are we going to get the data, monitor/validate the data, and review/clean/verify the data? We went from the traditional data capture modality (see Figure 6.1) where the patient had to travel to various locations and the site staff was responsible for entry into the electronic health records (EHRs), as well as the EDC and supporting the

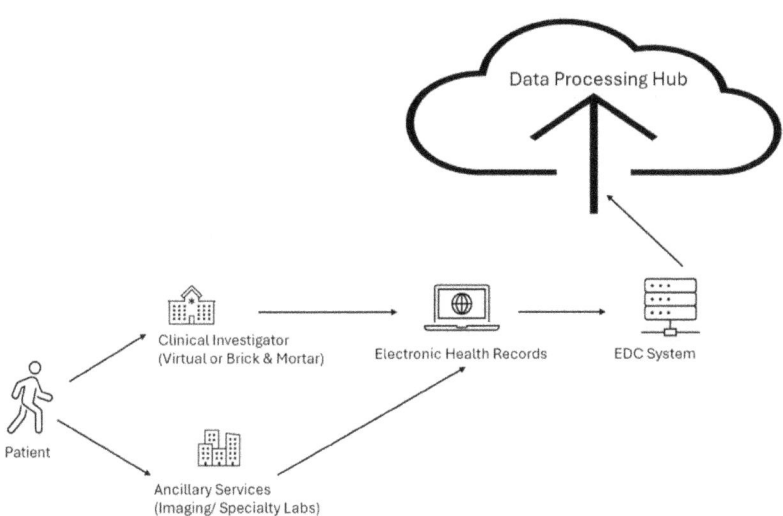

FIGURE 6.1
Traditional data capture model.

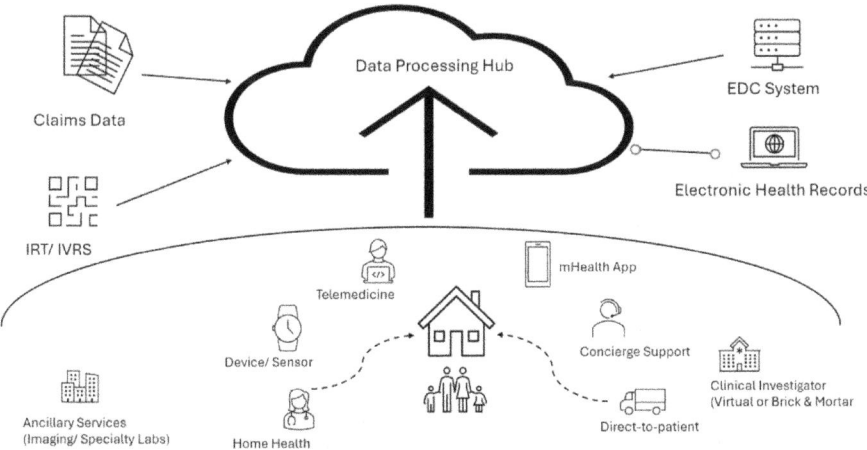

FIGURE 6.2
Data flow in a DCT setting.

coordination of results for the ancillary services. The CDM is responsible for multiple reconciliation points and, along with the CRA, ensuring that transcription errors are not causing issues in cleanliness of the data.

Now if we look at how the data flow changes in a more decentralized capacity (as shown in Figure 6.2), you will see there is a more streamlined experience for patients and the trial components are brought to them versus the traditional model where the patient is responsible for more of the navigation approach. From a CDM perspective there are many additional sources of data, the potential need for additional reconciliation points, and more reliance on smart programming and validation checks than the traditional model.

Now What?

Now that we are post pandemic and authorities have seen the positive outcomes of the approach to decentralized elements, where do we head from here? The likely outcome will be more hybrid trials and providing optionality to patients. Additionally, the term of DCTs will likely start to fade from use. We have talked about decentralized elements being more important and prominent than decentralizing a full trial. With that in mind we will likely start to see terms like modernized trials and patient-centric trials. What does this mean for our CDM staff? More likely than not it means that the talent that is needed will shift.

Analytical thinking will become a core component of what is needed in our CDM staff moving forward. These individuals will need to be able to dig into the why of the data rather than just reporting on it. In addition, CDMs as always will need to keep in mind that bigger picture – looking outside of the primary data collection and assessing additional data that can triangulate a larger picture of the patient's overall care.

How do we get to that larger picture? We need to look at the type of data to determine where we start. There have traditionally been two types of data – site data and patient data.

- Site Data – this is data that the site collects, transcribes, or helps support the transfer of to the data handler. Examples of site data include CRF data, laboratory data, and safety data.
- Patient Data – this is the data that the patient collections/provides in the form of direction collection. Examples of patient data include consent and eCOA/ePRO.

There is a shift now to also take the site and patient data and look at it from a slightly different angle: active data versus passive data collection.

- Active data – this is data that is collected directly through interactions with patients and site. Examples of active data include eConsent, ePRO, and question completion on CRFs.
- Passive data – this is data that is collected without direct interaction with patients and sites. Examples of passive data include claims data, data collection from consented wearables, and/or sensors.

As we shift to the addition of passive data collection there is a need for the risks associated with that passive collection to be shared with all study participants (patients, sites, sponsor, and data handlers).

When we put all these four elements together to build that bigger picture, it requires foresight in terms of deciding which data needs to be captured at the source, selecting between active and passive approaches, as well as possible ramifications for the CRF design. In addition, there will be consequences for the data review approach depending on which way data collection will be implemented.

Let us go a bit further into this in the next section.

Are DCTs Really the Way of the Future?

There is not a "one size fits all" approach when it comes to DCTs. The future of the trial paradigm is definitively changing. The concept of bringing trials to where the patients are will continue to be a focus for the future. So, where do we begin? The best first step is to assess a protocol to see if it is optimal for decentralized elements.

As we often hear, the best place to start is with the end in mind. It is always optimal to start a study with the decentralized elements as part of the start-up, especially from a data management perspective. There are times though when this isn't possible as decentralized elements are utilized to support poor enrollment and retention within a study. This creates a mid-study change for the CDM staff, and previous elements need to be taken into consideration.

The next element to consider is project risk evaluation. When performing a risk evaluation, the CDM should be included. Remember to bring forward questions about the decentralized elements, technology, and patient oversight. Some of those questions may be as follows:

- Who oversees the patient safety during a remote visit?
- Has the technology platform been validated by the sponsor?
- How is the data being stored and transferred for the decentralized elements?
- What happens to the data if there is a lack of compliance with the decentralized elements?

This then brings us to the next consideration, protocol adherence. CDMs are often responsible for helping to identify protocol violations or deviations. The implementation of automated platform-based checks can further ease the burden when looking at patient-collected data. This assists the patients and aids them with what is next without leading them to a particular response.

While the data is being captured in a more real-time capacity it bears the question of who is responsible for the oversight of the patient and how quickly. Real-time availability of data not only means that sponsors have access to data more quickly but also means that there is a responsibility to review that data in a more real-time manner. This can fall to the medical monitors, remote patient monitoring center, or the investigator depending on the criticality of the data. We will discuss the idea of remote patient monitoring and potential impacts a bit later.

An additional consideration that is often not thought of is the technology burden. How many different tools, systems, and platforms are we asking not just patients to interact with but also the site staff and CDMs. Each of these elements requires validating from a CDM perspective, training from a site and patient perspective and support for all three end user groups. While it might be cool and fun to implement a wearable, if there is no comfort with the technology the physician/site won't enforce compliance, the patient won't use it, and the CDM won't have data from it. Neglecting to take this into consideration will lead to a failure on collection of necessary data for the study endpoints, even if just exploratory in nature or for a subset of patients.

The final element of consideration, which is probably the most crucial in the CDM's mind, is data quality. As we shift from traditional brick and mortar site-collected data toward primary source capture (direct from patient capture) there may be a shift in the quality of the data. The advantage of primary source data is that it does allow programmatic alerts and notifications in a more real-time capacity. Ultimately, this can improve the quality of the entire study data as it can catch "problem" earlier and allow for corrective action earlier.

Successful DCT Execution Example

Let's look at a successful decentralized clinical trial and review how and why it was deemed a success. It was right before the COVID-19 pandemic, and the trial had been originally designed to be conducted in a fully decentralized capacity. Sites would screen patients using their EMRs. The patients would then be invited to participate in the study by email, portal, phone call, or when they happened to visit their physician. Patients were directed to a website to learn of the trial and if they were interested, they were able to opt in to be screened.

Once the patient had been screened by the site's virtual coordinator and deemed eligible, the patient would download the mobile app and begin the eConsent process. The eConsent was conducted completely remote with the physician in a telehealth/telephone visit. Both electronic signatures were collected, and that patient was enrolled.

The study team worked with the drug depot to ship study medications directly to the patients, while keeping their identifying information confidential and separate from any study data. In addition to receiving the study medication directly to the home of the patient, there was also a wearable sensor sent for their utilization. Once both the study medication and sensor were received the patients were able to connect with support staff to walk through the setup process and answer questions they might have. The data was captured through the sensor, the mobile application, and patient claims data.

All of this was planned and set up prior to the pandemic hitting and as a result enrollment was not impacted by the pandemic. There were some additional positive results other than successfully completing the study. It was deduced that because of a completely decentralized study and allowing the study to fit into the patient's life, reducing burden, there was an almost even gender distribution among those patients. The patient population traditionally observed in clinical trials is white, male patients. Consistently underrepresented are women, the elderly, and people of color.

Additionally, the diversity of the patient population reflects that of the indication being studied. This is something that has historically been an issue and is now being added as a mandate for all phase III studies moving forward.

The credit for the success of this study should go to the study team. They worked through the project risk evaluation plan, developed data flows from both a site and patient perspective, and determined where additional support and touch points would be needed to help retain patients while reducing site staff burden.

DCT Execution Example – Room for Improvement

As previously mentioned, not all protocols should be delivered in a completely decentralized capacity and the learning of what works and what doesn't is continuing to grow. The next example I would like to dive into is an example of a well-intended, but less successful, fully decentralized study.

Again, this protocol started off being written in a completely decentralized capacity. The patients would find out about the study through social media, ads, and promotional websites. The patients would pre-qualify themselves and click on interest in the study. Once they completed the pre-qualification that centralized investigator and support staff would reach out to the patients.

This was the first failure point. Patients were not known to the centralized investigator and likely more importantly, the centralized investigator was not known to the patients. The patients would not answer the phone or outreach from the virtual site or the centralized coordinating center. This would lead to a large dropout. Quickly the study staff learned that the top of the funnel needed to be much larger than originally anticipated.

To help alleviate the issue with identification of "real patients", the virtual investigators turned to their EMRs to start finding the right patient population and reaching out to known individuals. The next step was obtaining consent. The consent process was relatively smooth in that the patient and physician were able to go into a meeting and review the protocol and sign the consent.

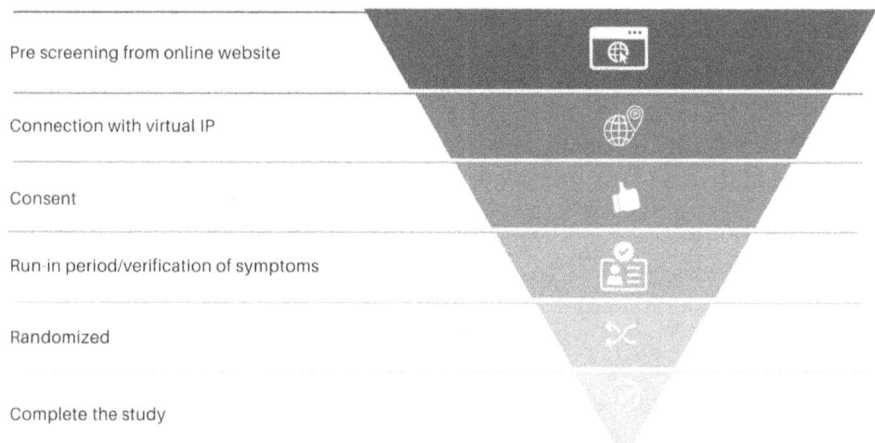

FIGURE 6.3
DCT recruiting and patient interaction funnel.

The only slight flaw with this step was the number of technologies that were needed as the platform used for consent was a different platform than that used for consent. This required both the patient and physician to be relatively savvy in having multiple browser windows open at once. Additional hurdles occurred when one or both of those technologies failed, in which case support was needed, thus delaying the process. This would require rescheduling both the patient and physician, pushing out the timeline for the consent and causing a loss of interest.

The next step was going through the run-in period and verification of compliance with medication and symptom collection. The direct-to-patient shipments went off without any incidence and were handled through the depot in a similar manner as the first example; patient-identifying information was stored in a separate area from the study data. The recording of symptoms on the diary was a bit more problematic. The platform chosen for the study was web-based and not app-based. The time that it would take to access the system to record symptoms (which needed to be recorded 24 hours a day) and the way in which the data was saved made analysis of the data difficult and compromised the quality of that data.

The third step was randomization. Because of the difficulties of data capture for the run-in period, it led to a large dropout rate prior to randomization as their symptoms did not qualify them for the study. There could have been several root causes for this:

- Patients misreported in the initial self-assessment the severity of their symptoms and should never have been screened

- The chosen platform made entry difficult and unclear and caused misreporting of the symptoms
- The back end of the data was not clear on the timeframe for capture and analyzing who qualified was not as accurate as it could have been

Again, this presented a large challenge with a larger than anticipated drop-out and the necessity to continue the pre-screening process.

Eventually, the study team broadened the outreach and were able to screen and filter through the process the appropriate number of patients to complete the study. After the database was locked and analysis started, additional issues arose. Some of the data records were not extracted completely, data points of capture were not easily deciphered, and ultimately when analysis was finished the study failed to prove the endpoints were met.

So, was this an issue of the protocol? An issue with the enrollment of the right type of patients? Or did technology fail the study? In my opinion, it was a case of all three – the perfect storm of what could go wrong in a study.

If we review both case studies, there are several lessons to learn from them and to keep in mind for future projects.

- CDM needs to be part of the planning process from the beginning
- It is important to ensure that the site and patient are kept in mind when developing data and patient journeys
- Data management is data management – there aren't as many differences between decentralized elements and traditionally captured data
- The review of data will fundamentally be the same with a slight mindset shift when the source of the data shifts
- Picking the right decentralized elements and tools for implementation is key to successful execution

Let us review each of these a bit further and determine what changes for CDM in a DCT setting.

What Changes for CDM in a DCT Setting?

When looking at the CDM process, let's start at the beginning. We discussed previously the risk evaluation. While this is a vital step and the DM team should be involved, there are other steps at an organization, not necessarily at the project level, that should be part of the early planning. This would ensure that the technology vendors chosen are validated, the specifications and requirements are clearly documented, and those elements are kept in mind when applying a decision to the study.

The best practice at the beginning of each study is to develop a patient and data journey. The patient journey should show the benefit of the addition of decentralized elements and evaluate the impact it will have on the sites at the same time. From a data perspective, a best-practice approach is a test transfer of data. This is especially important if the data is primary data and there is no source to verify it against. This gives the DM team an early understanding of the format, the quality, and ability of analysis as the study continues to collect data. Knowing where all the data points come from, the frequency of transfers should be included in the data journey.

The fundamentals of data management apply to decentralized studies in the same manner as a traditional on-site study. The 5 Vs of data science come to mind when thinking about the principles applied.

- Volume
- Velocity
- Variety
- Veracity
- Value

The volume of data as mentioned previously in Chapter 2 will vary based upon phase, size, and therapeutic area; however, it may not differ based upon whether the trial is a traditional or decentralized trial. The real impact will be the source of the data.

A key example would be the inclusion of a sensor that captures data in real time. An example of this is an actigraphy sensor. These types of sensors capture data at a microsecond frequency, looking at data points such as steps, exertion, and gyroscopic location. Suppose we look at the math, that is 8.64×10^{10} or 8.64 E + 10 or 86,400,000,000 in a single day, for a single data point. If we are now collecting multiple data points as mentioned earlier, you see the volume quickly becomes overwhelming. There is no way a human alone can review this volume of data, so we will need a shift in how the data is processed, consumed, and curated.

The velocity of data, however, may be beneficial for human review, as it represents more timely and, therefore, more valuable, data. One of the big differences is that in a decentralized trial data may come in faster than in a traditional study with the implementation of sensors and real-time data captured at a patient's home at the exact time of the visit. Historically this visit data has been captured on a source document and later transcribed into a case report (whether paper or electronic).

The variety of data will likely be similar between decentralized and traditional studies. There is nothing to say that a traditional trial won't have the same elements as a decentralized trial. However, with more complex study designs and our attempt to gather more data in a single protocol, we notice that the number of data types and vendors associated with that data increases drastically over the last few years.

The veracity of the data will likely be more uncertain in a decentralized trial when a larger volume of the data is patient-reported or captured in a remote way that may or may not have source documentation that isn't in the database itself. Again, referring to Chapter 2, this is where the power of the audit trail may become even more important. The larger the volume of data and the velocity to which it is being consumed, the higher the benefit of reviewing not just the data itself but also the audit trail of that data – specifically, where and when the data was originally captured for that patient-collected data points. It isn't that we don't trust our patients; it is more of a question of whether the data accurately reflects what was being asked in the timeframe it was being asked.

Finally, the value of the data could be considered the same across the two types of trials; however, there may be more "noise" in the value in a decentralized trial. The example given above of an activity tracker is a good one. Is there value in having every microsecond worth of data? Can a daily summary suffice? What is really needed to meet the endpoint?

Real-Time Data and Remote Patient Monitoring

Another area that will change in the DCT setting and have a drastic impact on data is the concept of real-time data and remote patient monitoring. Real-time data collection is exactly what it sounds like: collection of data in real time, delivered immediately after the point collection (though it is important to mention that real-time data is not the same as dynamic data). Real-time data collection can lead to the expectation of real-time data processing and real-time data review. Is there value in this and what would that mean to staffing of an organization?

Sounds like a large expectation. Think back to the wearable sensor data example before and let's expand upon that.

- $8.64 \text{ E} + 10$ in a single day for a single data point
- Scientists have found an average person can process 74 gigabytes of data per day ($\sim 5.92 \text{ E}+11$ bits)
- It will take approximately one human, one day to process a single patient's wearable data for a single sensor
- Assume the study involves 1,000 patients and runs for 24 months

With the above figures, it is clear that a company would need *1,000 employees for 2 years* to review just that single type of real-time reported data. When is the last time anyone was able to get 1,000 people to work on supporting a study of this size? This doesn't seem an effective or efficient utilization of resources. This leads to the first case of setting expectations on the real-time review of data.

The second concept of remote patient monitoring examines the type of data being collected and delivered and the expectation of the level/role of individuals reviewing that data. A good example of this is a heart monitor.

Often heart monitors are used to remotely collect cardiac safety data for patients. What isn't often seen is the expectation that the CDMs review and make medical decisions on patients based on that data. I don't know about you, but I would not want to be responsible for monitoring cardiac data and making recommendations without a medical degree. Typically, there are cardiac safety monitoring centers to support this type of review.

The review is real time with the support of alerts and range notifications. What is not done though is direct outreach to patients that there is an issue with, and that action may be needed immediately. These centers don't have access to patients; they reach out to the physicians who aren't always available during extended hours and decisions on the care of the patient will still ultimately fall to the physician. Why should that expectation change because the data is being collected for clinical research? This leads to the second case of setting expectations on the remote patient monitoring expectations and appropriate individuals involved in that review.

The Introduction of Artificial Intelligence (AI)

"Artificial Intelligence", two of the most dreaded words in clinical research that might instill fear around job security to CDMs. It is crucial, however, to understand that AI alone will not be able to replace the work that CDMs have been successfully performing for years. Rather, AI is intended to support and ease some of the manual burden that CDMs have faced over the years.

As we discussed earlier, the volume of data is continuing to increase with the complexity of trial designs and additional external sources of data. With this the need for AI and enhanced processing tools becomes more necessary. In addition, a more powerful processing engine will allow for the CDM team to more effectively and agilely move the data through the study life cycle. With the support of AI, the expectation is for additional ability to scale data collection, allow flexibility in collection methods, and enhance the intelligence that is applied to review that data.

This got me to thinking about my past as a CDM. I remember when I first started in the industry reviewing a dataset. I first started by doing an A-to-Z sort of the data. I looked for outliers, identified those patients, and put it into an Excel file. Then I would look for trends with that patient and put that in the Excel file. Next, I would look for trends across that site and put those in the Excel file. Finally, the tricky part – did any of what I documented mean anything? Was there anything noticeable that should trigger a query to the site? These fundamental steps were my attempt at classifying, cataloging, sorting for quality, and checking for integrity.

How could AI have supported my efforts above? Let's look at the fundamental steps and how they may have changed:

1. Classifying – utilizing AI would have enhanced the speed and volume of areas that could be classified for the data. It could classify data by type, location, and input, for example.

2. Cataloging – every step that I took I tracked manually in an Excel file. With AI cataloging and ensuring traceability of data would be a significantly more efficient task. Additionally, with the increased number of imports and areas where data is stored, AI can expedite the process and cataloging of the necessary data.

3. Quality – AI can enhance the speed for some of the easy, low-hanging data errors. Looking quickly the machine can determine if there is duplicate data, or if there is illogical data and then help support the prevention of these in the future (enhancing system features to not allow these types of errors)

4. Integrity – this may be the area where AI has the largest impact and benefit. Allowing AI to support the creation of the master data file across multiple sources and ensuring that the other steps above have been done and documented. This step for an entire company's worth of data could have such a large impact that it may save even years of time from the manual approach that previously existed.

The aforementioned enhancements are impressive and beneficial, sure. But AI can't do it all. There will always remain the need for the human element in clinical research. What can't AI do without human oversight or input and will remain human-centric, at least for a little while longer?

- Creation of data strategy
- Creation of data culture
- Calibrating devices and sensors
- Creating data governance
- Determine business requirements, determining organizational needs
- Pursuing security incidences and escalations to appropriate authorities

Utilizing AI will enhance our capabilities to draw early insights into data, patient safety, and overall effectiveness of the data collection methods.

Summary

The past several years seem to have warp-sped the advances in data collection in clinical research. When we look at the evolution:

- 1747, Jame Lind conducted the first controlled clinical trial of the modern era

- 1800s, placebo first appears
- 1943, the first double-blind controlled trial is performed
- 1964, Declaration of Helsinki
- 1990s, introduction of Electronic Data Capture
- 2011, first decentralized trial conducted
- 2013, FDA introduced eSource guidance document
- 2019/2020, COVID-19 data collection changes recommended
- 2023, FDA introduces DCT guidance document

The initial advances in clinical research and the associated data collection for it were very slow in comparison to some of the recent changes and updates seen in the 21st century.

Reflecting on the topics in the chapter, DCT has changed the clinical research environment and while we are not currently in a pandemic shutdown, those changes are here to stay. We looked at a successful example of a fully decentralized trial and one that had areas for improvement. The drug development industry can benefit greatly from sharing of case examples similar to above so that all can learn and progress the way we deliver trials to patients and collect the necessary data to deem the products of the future safe and effective treatments.

While I can't guarantee that full DCTs will be the way of the future, and in fact don't see that being the case, the key take away is offering options to patients and sites based upon the study, patient population, and region of the research. Many of the decentralized elements have been piloted by sponsors. The next step is determining when the pilot process stops and an increase in utilization occurs. How do we ensure that there is comfort and confidence in the execution of these decentralized elements? Data – validated, reliable and quality data – will help drive the adoption of these elements.

As reflected in the final topic we discussed the changes necessary for clinical data managers as decentralized trials evolve the clinical research paradigm; it is important to remember that there is still a vital need for CDMs. DCTs have taught our CDMs that they are needed now more than ever with a larger volume of data and the velocity of which it is being consumed in. While there is definitively a need for the day-to-day operational review, tasks are shifting. With the introduction of AI and advanced analytics, CDMs are shifting their responsibilities from traditional data management into the data science role. Let us explore in the next chapter how we, as expert clinical data managers or emerging new talent, can truly make change by finally stepping out of the shadow.

7

Stepping Out of the Shadow

With the complete set of CDM knowledge in our back pockets now and having obtained a glimpse of what the future holds for the CDM profession, this last part of the book is dedicated to focus on you and how to boost your career and impact within your respective area.

We will do this by sharing real-life examples, looking at certain soft skills to focus on, and helping you to identify situations that present opportunities to step out of the shadow.

Even if you are somebody who is perfectly happy in your current role and have no real desire for a change or career progression, this chapter will still be valuable, when it will not be you but the company or the evolution of our profession to force the change on you.

So let us explore the following puzzle pieces and try to put them together to form the more complete vision of how we can help our company, clinical research, and ultimately ourselves, by identifying and acting on the opportunities that surround us.

- Embracing accountability
- From back seat passenger to co-pilot
- Working cross-functionally
- Time to show off

Embracing Accountability

There are many CDM deliverables that are on the critical path during the execution of clinical studies or regulatory submission activities. Let us use two of the key CDM deliverables: a) building the clinical database and b) Locking the clinical database, as examples of how embracing accountability for these milestones is a crucial first step toward showing the value of CDM and earning trust and respect from your colleagues in other functions.

DOI: 10.1201/9781003648314-7

Let me set the stage with a very familiar scenario, which is unfortunately not an exception but the norm. Starting with the clinical database build example, we do know that a CDM starting point for this activity is the existence of a, not necessarily final, yet robust, clinical protocol outlining the schedule of events and defining the clinical data domains to be collected. In my experience these 3–4 months before the overhyped milestone of FPI are quite intense for the entire team, especially for our colleagues in clinical operations. The company's focus lies on finalizing the protocol, identifying and initiating clinical sites, getting the regulatory documentation in place, and working with the PIs to start identifying suitable patients.

It seems to be assumed as a non-negotiable given mandate that within this flurry of activities CDM must, to name just a few of the more prominent items,

- Build a clinical database, with hundreds, if not thousands of edit checks
- Ensure adherence to data standards
- Build integrations with other data sources, such as RTSM (Randomization and Trial Supply Management)
- Perform validations and UAT
- Deliver the analytics tools to perform RBQM activities

To make things even more challenging, we have to remember that at this stage of the clinical study, more often than not, protocol changes will happen, new data sources will be added last minute, and a medical monitor might request a deviation from the agreed-upon standard; however, the timeline for CDM to deliver a robust database will not be adjusted by pushing out the FPI date to accommodate for the extra work needed.

So, what can we do in this very typical scenario, if we are the DD, CDSL, or Head of the CDM Team?

Let me start by mentioning what NOT to do by including a character trait and mindset that never leads to a positive outcome for anybody involved.

I am talking about Passive Aggressiveness and a mindset of "this is not my fault and there is nothing I can do about it". Trying to be even clearer, the more important issue with the "Passive Aggressiveness" is not necessarily the "Aggressive" part, but the "Passive" part.

What do I mean by that? Regardless of which CDM role I am representing in this scenario, taking on a passive approach, possibly even extending into the sentiment of being a victim of the circumstances, will not benefit the delivery at hand, the study team, or the reputation of the CDM department.

Multiple proactive and ongoing actions should be driven by the CDM representatives in preparation and delivery of the clinical database build. These are:

- Open and continuous communication with the study team, by ensuring CDM deliveries are part of the meeting agenda.

- Clearly state the status of progress and outline possible risks such as resourcing, complexity, unexpected changes, and vendor issues.

- While outlining the risks, it is important to always add the remediations put in place by you and/or your team.

- And most importantly, remember that you and your team represent the subject matter expertise for the task of building the clinical database and taking care of external data sources. It is on you to earn a level of trust from the rest of the study team by showing that you are embracing accountability for this delivery.

- No excuses, no finger pointing, not being an alarmist, but clearly guiding and leading the way through open communication, outlining risks and offering solutions.

Moving on to the second example, which represents arguably the most significant and visible CDM delivery – the clinical database lock.

Still to this day, I see so many companies implementing "Data Review Meetings" or "Database Lock Meetings" that are run by Clinical Operations or Project Management. To emphasize again, the individual representatives of those functions are most often outstanding professionals with the best intentions at heart; however, leading the data review journey and deciding when a database is ready for lock are and should not be part of their job description.

To illustrate why, I can share the following real-life examples with you.

A mid-size Biotech company which had engaged with the CRO I was working for, had engaged with my CDM team for a good number of late-stage oncology studies. This Biotech company had a few in-house CDM professionals liaising with my team. It became apparent very quickly that the relationship between those CDM professionals and the rest of the team on the Biotech company's side was strained and lacked trust and understanding of their abilities.

The Biotech's CDM department had no real leadership and was part of a biostatistics-dominated biometrics group, which saw CDM as an inferior role and subservient to all other functions.

This resulted in Clinical Operations leading data review meetings and defining the database lock targets, with CDM being reduced to the role of executing queries not as a result of an objective IDRP, but from the subjective input of discussions between medical reviewers, CRAs, and clinical operations.

To make things worse, additional outside organizations were contracted to perform more data review tasks which were not directly mentioned in the IDRP. The result of this non-desirable set-up was multiple weekly meetings, with dozens of people, reviewing patient by patient manually and discussing what data issues deserved to be queried, and which ones were deemed to be acceptable.

Tied timelines, fractured relationships, and high frustration levels by many individuals resulted in the inevitable finger pointing to my CRO and their internal CDM representatives.

How could this scenario have been avoided?

Using my own advice, I am looking at what my own CRO CDM team and the CDM professionals at the Biotech company could have done differently first, rather than just pointing to the other functional groups.

Right at the beginning of the study, the combined CDM team from my CRO and the sponsor company had to form a stronger alliance, which did not happen. This is a common phenomenon when the sponsor representatives are new to an outsourcing approach and might be fearing for their own jobs, or, CDM approaches differ, and not enough time is invested to get on the same page right from the start.

Even more importantly though, the joined CDM team should have put in place proactively a "data review" or "data health status" meeting, inviting all other relevant functions, and should have led this meeting by literally and figuratively sitting at the head of the table.

In this meeting, the CDM lead, from either the CRO or the sponsor site, would report on items and metrics such as clean patient trackers, query status, and most importantly the data analytics from the risk review activities. These would then result in CDM assigning action items to:

- CRAs to follow up with clinical sites that are falling out of line for:
  - Not entering data quickly enough
  - Delayed query responses
  - Higher number of issues compared to other sites, suggesting a possible training need
  - Data changes after SDV, suggesting CRAs not performing SDV correctly
- Clinical Project Managers for:
  - Follow-up with external data providers such as Central Laboratories or ePRO providers, if they were not fulfilling their contractual obligations on data transfers
  - Ensuring CDM-related timelines were accurately reflected in the overall project management plan
- Medical Reviewers for:
  - Providing input on the robustness of the IDRP based on the medical review and oversight provided
  - Ensuring medical coding consistency through targeted review of all coded terms
- Biostatisticians and Statistical Programmers for:
  - Confirming smooth transformation from raw data to SDTM and ADaM datasets. Frontloading this activity avoids nasty surprises later on

- Ensuring continuous alignment between the objectives defined in the SAP and the ongoing review efforts, in terms of focusing on the "Critical to Success Data", that is, typically the data related to the primary and secondary endpoints of the study

A CDM-led data review meeting like this, implemented right from the start, would have built the foundation to trust CDM to lead the overall study team to the database lock. CDM could have ensured that additional resources joining the data review efforts would have been integrated, while adhering to the established IDRP, resulting in a truly objective and well-orchestrated database lock.

Not doing so created a "too many cooks in the kitchen" scenario, where there was no clear accountability for the review process, the data quality, and the database lock procedures.

In this real-life example, which is unfortunately more common than you might think, the data review meetings deteriorated even further, when even more technical items, such as freeze and lock procedures within the EDC system, were not decided by CDM, but in extensive meetings by leadership from the clinical and medical teams.

Wrapping up this particular example, it should not come as a surprise to you that the database lock got delayed by several weeks. The flow of new queries being generated did not seem to end. More and more parties wanted to look at the data to ensure that from their perspective it was correct. The guiding document, that is, the IDRP, became irrelevant, and the combined CDM team, which had never been in control of this delivery, was pushed more and more into the background by becoming the executor of the data decisions made by other functional representatives.

Trying to be fair, I find it understandable that in this case clinical operations representatives were trying to fill the gap to the best of their abilities. A gap that was created by the CDMs from the CRO and the sponsor not embracing the accountability right at the start for the tasks that should be led by CDM.

In this section we looked at the clinical database build and the database lock as two examples for when CDM professionals must embrace accountability to lead the rest of the team. "Leading" does definitely not mean to do it alone. CDM on its own would not be able to perform these tasks. It means to work cross-functionally and lead the joined team on these bumpy journeys toward the common goals.

In addition to the two aforementioned CDM deliverables that should be led by CDM, I want to mention:

- Creation and maintenance of the DMP with cross-functional input
- Creation, maintenance, and governance of the IDRP with cross-functional input

- CRF design, which goes hand in hand with database build activities
- Data Standards use
- Central monitoring of data for cross-functional risk assessments
- Vendor selections, for vendors that are clinical data providers (at lease for the data part)

Respect and trust are usually not just handed out. They need to be earned.

CDM professionals in lead roles, such as CDSLs, LDMs, Data Strategy Leads, or whatever name they might be given, need to have the endorsement from their respective leadership, SOPs to support this approach through unequivocally clear RACIs defining the accountable roles, and the confidence to rise to the challenge when duty calls.

From Back Seat Passenger to Co-pilot

Now that we have gone through a few examples of the importance of embracing accountability, let us look at other puzzle pieces to complete the full picture. In the previous section we looked at CDM-specific tasks. I would like to start this section by sharing a work-related example, which is not directly related to CDM, but illustrates how to step out of the shadow and recognize a situation that requires action and points to desirable soft skills that need to be developed over time.

The background to this example is as follows. In the early 2010s, I already had been the Head of CDM for a 1,200-employee Biotech company, as a Director, for a few years and I think it is fair to say that our CDM team, including my team, were respected for our quality work and subject matter expertise, in light of the fact that we played our part in the successful submission and approval of the first new Lupus drug in over 50 years.

Early in 2011, just before we got the approval from the FDA, we had one of our routine company-wide town hall meetings with our CEO and the entire staff, gathering in person in our auditorium. In these town hall meetings, the CEO would address the crowd, and you could ask questions through microphones, and the cameras would project your image on oversized screens and to other company locations for those who could not attend in person.

At this particular townhall the two VPs of Manufacturing and Sales/Marketing were asked to provide updates on progress for their respective areas in light of the expected FDA approval for our lupus drug.

The Sales/Marketing VP made it very clear in his presentation that his salesforce would be so successful in marketing and selling blockbuster drug, based on his analysis of the market, that demand would be so large that Manufacturing would not be able to keep up with demand.

The VP of Manufacturing in his very composed and less hyperbolic response outlined how he was maximizing the output of doses in creative ways and additionally how he was already working on expansions of staff and equipment to scale up to growing demands.

The back and forth between the two on stage was comical at times, but I am not sure if it was just my impression or others noticed as well that there was underlying tension building in positioning themselves and their team in front of the CEO and the entire company.

It culminated with both VPs agreeing to a bet of who would win this competition of either producing sufficient doses or selling more than we could get on pharmacy shelves.

Fast forward to the last townhall meeting of 2011 in December, just 10 months after the meeting where both VPs made that bet.

Despite receiving the great news of approval by the FDA in March of that year, the company struggled to sell it quickly enough due to different factors, such as pricing and the overall outreach strategy. In contrast to Sales/Marketing though, Manufacturing did a phenomenal job by even exceeding their highest production projections.

The lack of revenue and the unfavorable outlook for the coming quarters had negatively impacted on our stock price, and the CEO had announced the need for layoffs to keep costs down. These layoffs were planned for December and were hitting the Manufacturing team disproportionally high.

In this last town hall meeting of the year, the CEO tried to justify, in front of the understandably anxious crowd, the rationale to reduce staff. In my opinion, he was doing a very poor job, and his approach did not come across as sincere. It felt very unfair to me to punish the ones that had done such a great job in the manufacturing department.

My hand went up; I wanted the microphone. I didn't mind the 1,000+ people in the auditorium and the tense atmosphere. I felt that somebody had to say what was likely on the minds of most people in that room. Yes, my palms got sweaty, as the microphone usher got closer, but I felt I had the facts and employees' sentiments on my side.

As calmly as I could, taking deep breaths, I stood up and spoke the words that to this day make me proud to have spoken. I said

<CEOs first name>, my name is Michael Goedde, Clinical Data Management, my question for you is, how can it be that the Manufacturing team who clearly won the bet gets punished through layoffs, and the Sales/Marketing team who clearly lost the bet is being rewarded?

For one second or two there was an awkward silence. Then something amazing happened. Isolated groups of people started clapping and applause grew until almost everybody clapped.

I sat down and awaited the answer. It came in the, to be expected, corporate lingo.

Even though I might understand the underlying business rationale for the layoff move, the communication and execution of this move were atrocious, and the price was paid by colleagues who did not deserve this treatment.

Already on the way back from the auditorium to our respective offices, I was approached by many colleagues, some of which I did not even know until then, thanking me for saying what many people were thinking. Back in my office, our VP of Clinical Operations and my boss's boss provided positive feedback along the same lines.

Why am I sharing this story with you?

This chapter is about stepping out of the shadow and enhancing soft skills. I can assure you that when I had raised my hand to ask for a microphone to challenge the CEO's approach to justify the layoffs, I was not thinking "Michael, this is a great opportunity to step out of the shadow and try to make a name for yourself".

I was more driven by what I would hope becomes more common sense in terms of calling out actions and statements that are objectively questionable. Especially when words and actions are detrimental to a people-first and quality-oriented culture.

Interesting things happened after this town hall meeting to me. I found myself more often involved in either contributing or even leading cross-functional activities. I got promoted from Director to Senior Director of CDM, and when our company eventually got bought by a large pharma entity I was allowed to participate in some of the transition activities.

I do not know if those outcomes were a consequence or in any shape related to what had happened at the townhall meeting. However, I do want to believe that unintentionally showing my own CDM Team, my colleagues, and superiors that in addition to being a technical person and SME for CDM, that I cared for the wellbeing of the company and its people and was not afraid to speak my mind and did have something to do with the positive turn in my career.

Learning from this example, we can think about other opportunities in our work environment of how to move from a CDM backseat passenger to a Co-pilot role beyond CDM.

One key component is to look beyond the area of responsibility that we have in front of us. An LDM might primarily think about the next DMP that needs to be drafted for a given study, or a CDSL might be absorbed by the task of implementing an appropriate risk-based approach. Regardless of the concrete task at hand, our general mindset should always be on:

- How does my deliverable impact colleagues in other functions?
- How can I improve the current process for this task I am doing?
- Can I make the work required from the functions preceding my task easier?

In addition to the items listed earlier, having a general understanding of where one's role sits in the overall chain of events at your company is important. It should allow you to think beyond your task and your area and allow for more opportunities to add value and expand your scope.

Backseat passengers do not ask questions or try to seek improvements. They follow the established routines, because "this is how we do things here".

Co-pilots, however, want to play a more leading and guiding role and be part of the group of people steering the company, your department, and yourself to success.

Let us look at more practical examples for you to try in your environment.

First you can look internally for opportunities to volunteer for initiatives or to work on cross-functional tasks. You might think that your current workload might not permit an extra hour per day to dedicate to another work assignment. This can certainly be true; however, trying to make yourself more valuable for the company and stepping out of the shadow will require some extra effort, at least temporarily.

In my experience, there are always opportunities to raise your hand to join:

- A process improvement initiative
- A standardization effort
- A task force looking at opportunities to automate manual processes
- A cross-functional team looking at reduction of redundant tasks between departments

Even though such tasks can create more working hours for you, they can be a welcomed break from your routine assignments.

A final thought on the topic of moving from passenger to Co-pilot, which I want to share with you, came in the form of a piece of advice I received from the aforementioned VP of Operations at that Biotech.

She and I had sporadic catch-up and feedback sessions. In one of those sessions, I asked her for advice on how to prepare myself eventually for more influential roles and if I ever would have the chance to achieve VP levels.

In her response, she was candid as usual. She pointed out how my technical background, subject matter expertise, and overall soft skills were indeed favorable toward loftier career goals, but pointed out a major obstacle for me, which would deny me future progress at any company.

Her key token of wisdom she shared with me, which remains vivid in my memory since the day she spoke the words, was "Michael, you have to transition from your predominantly tactical thinking to more strategic solutions and outlooks".

I recall leaving the meeting slightly confused, because I did not fully understand the difference between thinking tactical versus strategic at that stage in my career!

At that point in time, I had been in the US for about 10 years and was a Director of CDM, had attended numerous conferences and workshops, but had not realized or understood that there was a difference between those two words. That same evening, I called, of all people, my father, who was a retired locksmith, but active in local community groups, to tell him about the feedback I got and asked him, if he had further insights. I do not think that he ever had to really think about such questions throughout his career. Nonetheless, he did share, in my opinion, a surprisingly fitting sports analogy. He drew a distinction between the tactical measures sports teams implement to either countermeasure or exploit specific strengths or weaknesses of the opposing team in a given game. However, in contrast to the tactical direct approach in a game or even in set play, there is the strategic approach of a team representing their overall philosophy of play envisioned by their coaching staff for entire seasons.

A stroke of genius from my dad!

So many learnings that can be derived from the combined input from a global industry veteran, like that VP of Operations, and my retired, often grumpy yet well-intended blue-color background Dad.

Concretely, when I think about the career evolution from tactical to strategic, I see:

- Moving from tactical to strategic approaches being similar to advancing from being the player in a team, with a specific task, to becoming the team's captain or coach
- Even as a brilliant player, developing the understanding of how one's specific skill set and talent fit into the bigger picture and mission of the team and overall organization
- The shift of the time horizon, where for tactical goals the mission can be accomplished within a short period of time, because the "goal line" is in sight, whereas the strategic goals will often require multiple tactical steps from numerous participants over longer periods of time to show the desired outcome
- More figuratively speaking, it means standing up and looking over your cubicle walls, opening your office door and stepping outside, with the purpose of understanding what is going on outside of your CDM role you are fulfilling for a given study
- Asking yourself of how tactical tasks, such as the line of code you are writing, the database you are designing or about to lock, the clinical data you are reviewing, or the conference you are attending, fit into the overall strategy of your team, department, and company

I strongly believe that understanding the difference between tactical and strategic approaches, and knowing when to apply them, is a fundamental building block for making more meaningful and noticeable contributions in your work environment and increasing the likelihood of upward career movements.

Remembering that VP of Operations, Ann Wang, who unfortunately passed away too young in 2017, leaving a legacy of memorable clinical research work, and a generation of inspired individuals, me being one of them, who continue to benefit from the wisdom she shared.

Working Cross-Functionally

Moving on to other aspects and considerations of CDM stepping out of the shadow.

We have already seen multiple references and a few examples around cross-functional engagements.

The familiar phrases around "It takes a village to . . ." or "There is no 'i' in Team" also apply to clinical research. It takes hundreds of professionals from dozens of backgrounds and specialty areas to bring a new drug to market.

I want to share with you a few additional examples of how it does not only benefit your CDM department or yourself, but, more importantly, the actual purpose of our industry, which is to bring more effective and safer medicinal products to the market.

By now, we have hopefully solidly established the understanding of the pivotal role reliable clinical data takes in clinical research and CDM's overall accountability for this task.

Important to understand, though, is that similar to most CDM professionals who are likely not having any meaningful background or understanding of, for example, the manufacturing process of a new experimental drug and the difficulties of its synthesis, other professions look at the CDM area without a clue of what we actually do.

Let us stay with the manufacturing example. For us in CDM, what we actually care about in this regard is that our manufacturing colleagues deliver sufficient experimental drug, on time and with reliable storage and shipping information, in order to not delay the start and execution of our clinical studies. We want to respect their expertise, and it is a given that at the appropriate times they represent their area of expertise and accountability in cross-functional team meetings.

Through these interactions, they, meaning manufacturing, will over time establish a reputation of trust and reliability, or if deliverables fail short of expectations, steer discussions on how manufacturing is in disarray, may need help, or consider replacements and outsourcing options.

What does this mean for CDM? It means that in contrast to functions such as clinical operations, project management, regulatory affairs, and medical directors, which are considered industrywide, a given within a clinical study team, CDM, in many places, must make itself heard.

Similar to Manufacturing, our pre-requisites and final deliverables rely on other functions' input. This input needs to be provided on time and be on point to allow CDM to execute with excellence.

However, in the same way we in CDM likely do not have the understanding of what Manufacturing's input needs are and how complex their work is, and how we only see the final product, we in CDM have to proactively speak up and make our cross-functional needs clear.

Examples of CDM cross-functional input needs include the following:

- Early access to protocol synopsis or early draft to understand and plan for scope of study at hand, as well as having the opportunity to provide input on clinical data to be collected
- UAT from CRAs during the database build process
- Creation of the central piece of clinical data review – The IDRP
- Creation of the DMP
- Centralized Monitoring, that is, collaboration with clinical operations on risk-based approaches related to site management
- Database lock activities

Even though these examples may seem like a given to us in CDM, I can assure you that they are not common practices at many companies.

I will provide reasoning and a possible solution for this disconnect now. For colleagues or people in general who are outside of CDM, we continue to be mostly a black box and hard-to-grasp profession. I am sure many of you CDM professionals reading this have tried different approaches to explain to outsiders what it actually is what you are doing, and got the polite, yet puzzled look of pretending to understand on their faces.

The same is true for many of our colleagues at work. In most cases they do know what they actually expect from CDM, meaning an on-time delivered EDC database, "squeaking clean" data, and a flawless database lock at the end.

There is a knowledge gap, not meant in an accusatory, but more in an understandable matter of fact way, and it is on us in CDM to make every possible attempt to bridge the relevant pieces of this gap.

These are:

- Clarify timing and scope of the required input for CDM to have successful, high-quality, and on-time deliverables
- Share the complexities and risks of some of the required steps and how CDM will be addressing them
- When possible, share the relevance of your approach and CDM's roles in general through references to regulatory guidelines, showing that this is not only your opinion, but your solution to comply with industry standards, regulations, and best practices.
- Through all your interactions, your goal is to leave your colleagues with the understanding that you are in charge and accountable of all CDM deliverables and will communicate transparently and candidly about:
  - Progress
  - Success

- Missteps and how to resolve them
- Action items you need done from other representatives
- Outlook on the next steps to be taken

Key takeaway for you is that in almost all cases that I have observed at companies, where CDM did not work proactively with other functions, did not embrace accountability, and did not bridge the knowledge gap, CDM gets pushed aside, becomes an afterthought, and ends up as the scapegoat for most of the delivery misses.

Even more damaging for CDM and the company, beyond a given study, is the long-term impact for all other studies and clinical programs at that company. Other functions will feel the need to fill the gap that CDM is leaving in their eyes, regardless of their perception being real or misconstrued.

Symptoms of such environments can range from project management taking on database lock planning, clinical operations leading clinical data review meetings, medical monitors deciding when a patient is clean and can be locked, all the way to the company deciding that CDM needs to be outsourced.

The last statement is only applicable to sponsor companies. Nonetheless, at full service CROs, the CDM gap can be seen as well, but in different areas.

For example, when business proposals are being prepared by the CRO through the business development team or the project manager and proposals team, for the interested sponsor company, without review and buy-in from CDM for CDM-related work.

Not understanding the CDM complexities to deliver high-quality outputs will lead intentionally or unintentionally to proposals not including the number of CDM hours truly required to deliver or requiring timeline shortcuts as crucial quality steps might be omitted.

I have personally seen too many examples of CRO representatives, due to their knowledge gap, who think of CDM and Biometrics roles in general, as the first area to cut hours, suggest shortcuts, and underestimate the complexity, with the sole purpose of achieving a more attractive pricing for the interested client.

Moving on to talk about how CDM can come out of the victim role and proactively put our best foot forward to avoid these situations.

Especially if you are already in a Managerial role or possibly Head of the CDM or Biometrics-related department, I found it very beneficial to volunteer for speaking slots at the department or town hall meetings of other functions. Examples of topics you can suggest to your counterparts are:

- Demystifying CDM
- Overview of CDM Deliverables
- Getting most value out of our clinical data
- Identifying study risks before they become a problem

These can then be 15–30-minute presentations, when you can position your department in the context of clinical programs.

I used this approach successfully at a few companies, about 3–4 months into taking over the position of Head of CDM. Yes, at the beginning you might sense some skepticism or disbelief; however, more often than not, I was met with a sigh of relieve, because our cross-functional colleagues were longing for somebody to step up and say "We CDM are accountable for these tasks, and we will ensure (with your support) to deliver".

Obviously, words need to be followed up with actions and you and your team will have to show an active presence in meetings, start leading CDM tasks, and deliver. Showcasing early successes will be important to further gain trust and boost confidence in your team.

Related to this first suggestion of you, or somebody from your team, presenting at other functional gatherings, it is also very beneficial, on the constant journey of breaking silos, to invite representatives of other functions to your own CDM meetings. To understand their needs, ask questions and build relationships.

Working cross-functionally does have benefits beyond running better clinical trials and having higher chances of success. It helps all involved individuals to expand their respective horizons and over time obtain a broader knowledge base, which will be required for higher level roles and executive positions.

Time to Show Off

Now that we have a) Embraced Accountability, b) Moved from Passenger to Co-pilot, and c) Started to work cross-functionally, we are ready to Show-Off!

When I say, "Show Off", I do not literally mean the annoying behavior of being a show-off and exuberantly promoting every CDM milestone. However, I do mean the achievement of culminating the journey from the back-office CDM mindset as an individual as well as a department and having morphed into a reliable powerhouse of excellence in CDM delivery. An environment where colleagues outside of CDM understand the value of our profession and engage with us on equal terms.

We are now part of the team!

People around you realize that high-quality clinical data does not happen by accident but is the result of dedicated hard work from professionals that can drive results. It represents the evolutionary step from the victim's mentality to becoming the master of our profession's destiny.

A few tangible examples for signs that can indicate that in your organization CDM is where it is supposed to be and is adding maximal value:

- CDM presents or is mentioned periodically at global companywide townhall meetings
- Leadership sees value to increase CDM thought leadership by supporting conference attendance and board opportunities for organizations such as SCDM
- CDM is not seen as a commodity which can just be offshored to low-cost regions
- CDM is seen as a differentiating factor due to the main driver to gain maximum value in form of information from clinical data

In addition to these more tangible items, I also noticed that when things go well for CDM at a company, and the overall culture is conducive to a positive work environment, it will just feel right to you and the people around you.

When you and your team have stepped out of the shadow, I encourage you to spread the message to your colleagues in the industry. With new technologies and approaches there are always the lingering questions around the CDM profession going extinct. The very simple answer to this concern is that as long as there is a need for clinical data in our industry, there will be professionals to take care of it. I cannot think of better suited and qualified people than people with the CDM-Gene.

In summary, we have seen more examples of how to continuously evolve your department, your team, and/or yourself to position our work in a better and more truthful light.

The key take aways are to not shy away from embracing accountability for the role we ought to play in clinical research. Not embracing it is a recipe for disaster on all levels.

In this chapter we have learned how to pull ourselves out of the dark and help those around us to see us, respect us, and allow us to add significant value to our company.

I can assure you that trying out some of the suggestions from this chapter will dramatically improve CDM's reputation and perception in your company . . . ., if the company is mature enough to allow it and has the appropriate culture in place.

With this confidence booster in place, we can now move on and change the world. . . . By becoming an Industry CDS Advocate, which we will explore in the next chapter.

8

Becoming a Clinical Data Science Advocate

You will have realized by now that the profession of CDM is constantly evolving. Starting from the fundamental building blocks that we established in the earlier chapters and gaining the understanding of what good and robust CDM looks like, we will now venture into the areas of how to continue to push the CDM value throttle all the way.

In the previous chapter we looked at "stepping out of the shadow" from a more individual point of view, whereas now we will expand into the realm of organizational and industry areas of influence and advocacy.

This does not mean that this chapter is only intended for established department heads or industry leaders of CDM. We will share examples of how to start the journey toward becoming an advocate and provide ways to further expand your areas of influence, when you have established yourself in your department, company and overall industry.

This chapter will also address a common misconception around possibilities of influence and advocacy any CDM professionals can have, regardless of their respective level or title. I have seen many cases of improved job satisfaction of people who see their actions having broader benefits than just completing the daily tasks at hand.

The goal over the next pages is to either awaken your desire to take the first step toward making your voice heard or embolden you further by providing you with more examples and background on your advocacy journey you have already started. We will do so by looking at:

- Culture First
- What is the ROI for investing in CDM?
- How to measure and present success for CDM?

Culture First

It has become more frequent in recent years that senior representatives from Biotech, as well as large Pharma companies, have reached out to me to provide

 DOI: 10.1201/9781003648314-8

input on how to possibly improve different aspects of their respective CDM departments. These conversations often start by asking me about which technology vendor I would prefer for certain CDM areas, if I would prefer bringing CDM in-house compared to offshoring it, or, one of my " 'favorites", if CDM is better suited to sit *under* Biostatistics or Clinical. "Under!" Really? Haven't we learned anything in the last 20+ years?

My counterparts do react surprised when I tell them that most of their struggles are probably not related to the technology at hand or their operating model of CDM but rooted in the underlying culture of their company or specifically the culture within and toward the CDM department. When we then talk about a formal engagement of assessing gaps and areas of improvement, I do leave it unequivocally clear that we will go – Culture First!

To not lose sight of the aim for this chapter, which is describing the journey toward, and the characteristics of, a CDS Advocate, let us take this mental note – data Science Advocacy starts with advocating and leading the way toward the right culture.

What does it mean – right culture? How do we know when it is right or wrong?

Let us start with the more obvious and intuitive examples, which are not necessarily CDM specific, before moving to the more nuanced ones.

People First

Despite the high degree of technological penetration in clinical research in general, it is still humans who perform the key tasks of getting new medical breakthroughs to market. These humans will be more motivated to complete tasks within their work environment with the highest possible quality, ethical standards, and creative mindset, when they feel valued and treated with respect.

Even though common sense suggests that this should be the modus operandi in all organization, the unfortunate truth is that when executive leadership, especially on the C-suite level, lose their ethical north star and are only focused on maximizing profit margins; and when employees, under such leadership, change from being humans with a scientific background to a commodity with a number and a cost label attached to them.

These work environments are relatively easy to spot and should be called out by advocates of all backgrounds, because these companies and their respective leaders do not fulfill their original mandate and main reason of existence, which in our industry is to better human lives, but instead prioritize maximization of short-term profits.

Don't get me wrong. Businesses, in order to strive, drive innovation, expand their R&D investments, and fairly compensate their staff, have to be profitable. However, there are realistic and let's say more human and sustainable ways to grow, and there are unfortunately more ruthless approaches.

Symptoms of the less desirable work environments are:

- Environment of fear
- Mistrust
- Financial considerations take priority over quality
- Mistakes are being punished, rather than used as a learning opportunity
- Cultural events feel fake, forced, and disingenuous
- Managers and leadership in general tend to manage up, rather than support their own team
- Regular layoffs despite solid quarterly profits, which might just have been short of unrealistic goals, but still were better than the previous quarter or year
- Challenging the status quo or questioning (respectfully) the leadership is not welcomed

This list is much longer, but I am sure you get the picture and unfortunately might have already experienced, or are currently experiencing, some of the items above.

Emphasizing again, I am absolutely expecting and in full support for a clinical research company, be it a Pharma, Biotech, CRO, or technology company, to set challenging goals, drive excellence, and expect full commitment from their workforce. Having interacted and worked with 1000s of different clinical research professionals in all sorts of settings, I can say with confidence that the majority has chosen this industry fully embracing this challenge. However, what people have not signed up for is to serve misguided leadership in a toxic work environment that is not conducive to accelerating medical breakthroughs.

Let us take the previous items and circle back to the more specific area of data science advocacy. As an individual who wants to drive excellence in the clinical data space for your company, the foundation thereof is making people feel genuinely valued and empowered. With this cornerstone in place, it will be possible to create confidence and self-respect within the team, and more importantly, propagate and show the value of CDM cross-functionally.

Politics

The term "politics" is often used in the corporate setting, when people want to describe cultural aspects of a company related to:

- How to communicate with superiors and/or getting their approval
- The amount of red tape to cut through in order to be able to move ahead
- Emphasis on hierarchical structures and/or focus on levels and titles
- Approachability of leadership

- Leaders surrounding themselves with people who predominantly agree with them
- Infighting between departments or executives, rather than a One Team approach
- External image of the company does not represent the true sentiment of the majority of its workforce

Similar to the previous list, there are many more examples that people have in mind, when they refer to the politics of a company. Interesting though, in my experience, I have almost exclusively met people in the work environment who say that they are not interested in the politics of a company and do not want to get involved. They rather prefer to focus on their area of accountability and get things done, than wasting time and energy on items such as inflated egos, power grabs, or territorial battles for more influential positions.

Both cultural indicators, "People First" and "Politics", can be observed and felt rather quickly in companies. As an aspiring CDS Advocate and motivated professional, you will have to determine if there is a path forward and hope for the company in question to turn the toxic environment into a welcoming and prospering one. Depending on your assessment, you will have to decide to either step up and help this company to get out of its misery or stop wasting your precious time and energy at this place trying to fight the windmills of helping self-serving and margin-squeezing leaders to see the light.

Positioning CDM correctly in a company and demonstrating its far-reaching value are difficult tasks, even in well-run companies.

This brings us to the more nuanced cultural indicators.

As a reminder, our main goals as a CDS Advocate are:

- Ensure the unparalleled importance of reliable clinical data is understood throughout the organization
- Reliable clinical data is the result of trained CDM professionals, working diligently using state-of-the-art technology and efficient processes
- These CDM professionals must be empowered, trusted, and yes, held accountable, for all areas that touch on clinical data.

By looking carefully at these three items, we will recognize a few details mentioned within them, which are crucial success factors for sustainable success of any CDM organization, and indicators if your current work environment has room for improvement.

Let's analyze a few of them:

"Trained CDM Professionals" – the foundation of an exceptional CDM Team in terms of training, access to a network of experts and to reliable sources of industry's best practices comes for the most part through involvement at the appropriate conferences who relate directly or indirectly to the CDM

profession. Thus, I think that one key indicator of demonstrating if CDM is seen as a valued and differentiating department in a company is the support in terms of allocated budget to allow CDM staff to attend such events.

Unfortunately, I have seen, and still see, too many cases at companies where reasonable budgets for such events are not deemed essential or are disproportionally low for CDM compared to other functional areas.

A company where CDM leaders and regular staff are consistently deprived of the opportunity to interact with their peers in the industry, get exposure to the latest break-through technologies, or listen to inspiring key-note speeches should not be surprised to fall back into mediocracy, or worse, with regard to clinical data quality.

To balance out my previous statements a little bit, I fully understand that budgets are not limitless, and it cannot be a free-for-all in terms of conference attendance, which can be significant cost factor, taking into account the full costs around travel, accommodations, registration fees, and more. However, done correctly, such educational opportunities can be dosed in such a way that they do not break the bank and, at the same time, provide remarkable ROIs.

"State-of-the-art technology" – related to the previous item, which talked about developing and maintaining a well-trained CDM team, the same is true for the plethora of CDM-related technologies and the need to be up to date on available options and advancements.

First though, I want to draw your attention not to the technologies them-selves, but to the question of who is sitting in the driver's seat when it comes to evaluating and ultimately deciding on which technology to use for CDM. This is another indicator of the standing of CDM and prevailing culture at a given company. If CDM experts and/or leadership are only bystanders or just informed about which EDC, ePRO, data visualization, or analytics tool will be used, it should raise a few eyebrows.

Similar to most areas in CDM, even though accountability should rely within the CDM department, it always requires a cross-functional team to be successful. In the case of picking the right technology for CDM needs, input from areas such as IT, QA, Clinical Operations, Procurement, and pos-sibly other departments are necessary and welcomed. However, taking all cross-functional input and CDM's own subject matter expertise and experi-ence into account, it is ultimately the appointed CDM individual or team that should be able to articulate the reasoning for the decision to go for a given technology solution, and held accountable for the decision.

On the contrary, if CDM were to be not more than a bystander in such an initiative, it would be another indicator that the existing culture and outside perception of CDM's value is not conducive for building a differentiating and value-generating CDM department.

"All areas that touch on clinical data" – lastly, for this list, we will remind our-selves of the broad area CDM professionals have to cover and ask the ques-tion "Does CDM have (at least) a seat at the table for all these areas?" With

the background of all the previous chapters, we already know that beyond the default CDM assignments related to EDC-database builds, DMP creation, data review, and database lock, CDM's remit goes beyond and extends into:

- Protocol design
- Regulatory submissions
- Data Strategy for End-to-End clinical data flow
- RBQM
- Data Standards Management

To just name a few.

Therefore, when we have a closer look into cultural aspects at a given company, as they relate to CDM's integration into the cross-functional landscape, it is a good indicator if CDM is truly seen as, and empowered to be, the custodian of clinical data – or not. Concretely this means that SOPs and the way of doing business at this company should show that CDM professionals are entrusted to take on the lead role for CDM tasks and participate, by having a seat at the table, for all other areas that either use or can affect clinical data.

Concluding the "Culture First" part of this chapter, the key take home messages are to not only risk underestimating the importance of culture in a company, but also see culture as the bedrock for anything else that a company aims to achieve.

Within culture there are different aspects that can range from very obvious manifestations in terms of how staff is seen and treated, to the presence or absence of counterproductive political shenanigans, all the way to the more nuanced aspects we examined at the end.

CDS advocacy is therefore an extension of the advocacy for a people-first culture.

With this foundation in mind, we can now turn the page to the reality of business and explore how a fully integrated, respected, and striving CDM department can positively impact a company's performance and show a positive ROI.

What Is the ROI for Investing in CDM?

Investing in CDM is equivalent to investing in the effort of maximizing the level of efficiency and confidence to obtain reliable results of a clinical study that reflect the true safety and efficacy profile of an investigational drug.

Other operational functions play their critical roles as well and are essential to ensure successful study execution; however, it needs to be pointed out that ultimately it is the clinical data that has to "speak" the truth.

Let's look at the ROI discussion for CDM starting with some of the more frequent and basic occurrences. It is understandable that for many operational functions, and CDM not being an exception, the first thoughts around ROI in CDM will bring up the question of "Efficiency".

Examples of standard initiatives in CDM with the target of doing more with less are:

- Automation and reduction of manual process steps
- Use of Standards
- Streamline processes
- Identify and eliminate duplications of effort

Starting with the first one "Automation", CDM has many areas and opportunities to cut cycle times and deploy resources smarter through automation. Database design, data review, medical coding, third-party vendor ingestion, and reconciliation are just a few areas that are prime targets for CDM.

Taking on the role of a "Clinical Data Science Advocate", however, means not only ensuring the more basic and obvious areas of automation, but also to push beyond. Optimizing every process step through automation is just the start.

Key decision-making in CDM should also include extensive and governed use of Data Standards, with the expertise and instinct to find the right balance of strict enforcement, while addressing subjective preferences, but with enough flexibility to allow for meaningful exceptions for the rule.

If you are able to show in your respective work environment that one of the most prominent dimensions of any ROI discussion, that is, efficiency gain, has been optimized by the CDM team, and you can present the tangible benefits through objective KPIs, you will have set the foundation for more CDM value generation in your company.

Why? Well, with the efficiency component addressed and transparently monitored, your CDM team can build, implement, and demonstrate value creation for other ROI dimensions, such as quality enhancements, creating differentiating factors for the competitive landscape, cost optimization (to not use the word "cutting"), sales and marketing input, as well as nourishing a positive culture.

With this in mind, embracing the CDS Advocate Role means that beyond the daily execution of all CDM tasks, there must be a constant push and desire to explore CDM-driven initiatives that can hit as many ROI dimensions as possible, ideally crossing departmental barriers, real and perceived ones, to further strengthen the case to invest.

Let us consider a concrete example – in many companies, any sort of initiative, new technology, or activity that results in a Capital Expenditure (CAPEX) or Operational Expenditure (OPEX) will have to go through and approval process – rightly so. The approval process typically consists of the "Initiative Owner" presenting:

- The main reason for the initiative – what problem needs fixing?
- Industry landscape and benchmark data for current solutions
- Comparison between the status quo within the company and the desired outcome and new approach
- Required investment, that is, OPEX and CAPEX
- A timetable for key milestones and final delivery
- And, likely the most important part, the quantifiable ROI expectations

Let's take a slightly simplified example from a global CRO perspective, where the Head of CDM, who is also an avid advocate for promoting the standing of CDS, is convinced that establishing a sizeable Data Standards Team would be an important step for the entire company.

Preparing for the senior leadership approval committee meeting, this Head of CDM diligently prepares the ROI presentation by:

- **Explaining the Problem:**
  - Too many redundancies in the current process
  - "Reinventing the wheel" for items that are industry standards
  - Longer cycle times than competitors during the design periods, resulting in lost business
  - More frequent quality issues as staff has no access to established data standards
  - Painting the picture of the downside and consequences, if the initiative is not being approved
- **Industry landscape and benchmark data for current solutions:**
  - Presenting the regulatory mandate from the FDA to submit data in SDTM format, which underlines the need for data standards
  - Showing data of cycle time reductions comparing database builds using standards versus starting from scratch
  - Referring to publicly available and relevant white papers
- **Comparison between the status quo within the company and the desired outcome and new approach**
  - Average database build times shrinking from 12 to 7 weeks
  - 30% average reduction of effort during protocol amendments
  - Being able to provide a differentiating argument in front of prospective clients, when asked about innovative efficiency gains

- **Required investment, that is, OPEX and CAPEX**
  - OPEX: Hiring three FTEs, with one of them becoming the Global Head of Data Standards, and the other two being experts covering the different CDISC domains
  - CAPEX: Purchasing an established of-the-shelve data standards management systems that can integrate seamlessly into the current process
  - Presenting expected combined OPEX and CAPEX cost for Years 1–3 and estimates for the following years
- **A timetable for key milestones and final delivery**
  - Showing the timetable of the implementation, testing, and go-live dates. Pointing out that accountability to meet these milestones lies with the requestor – Head of CDM
  - Including financially relevant milestones such as breakeven point and expected growth trajectory for efficiency gains and new revenue streams
- **Quantifiable ROI expectations**
  - Creating a slow crescendo in the presentation with the intent of ensuring all decision makers understand not only the obvious need but also the additional potential.
  - Outlining first the undisputable efficiency gains for resourcing and manual steps
  - Following up with presenting examples around quality enhancements (e.g., reusing validated standards, instead of one-off solutions, or referencing recently released regulatory guidance, which promotes the use of standards)
  - And as a final push, presenting some unexpected benefits as well, which are: a) the creation of a new revenue opportunity in terms of offering data standards consulting and support; b) new marketing opportunities by adding a differentiating factor in client meetings; c) establishing new career opportunities for employees within Biometrics; and d) breaking down possible siloes in the company, by bringing functions together and rally behind a company standard for clinical data

The example stated earlier is actually not hypothetical. In one of the CROs that I served as Head of Global Data Operations, we had a four-people Data Standards Team, which needed a constant explanation for their reason to exist in the company. It was a repeating theme during cost cutting rounds to question that team's value. Therefore, we flipped the script and decided to stop playing defense and go into the offense, by asking for an increase in head count, despite being close to 0% utilization, investing in better technology, and bring data standards out from the basement and into the spotlight.

In return, we accepted the accountability to meet certain financial parameters related to an increase in billable work and actual business wins, as well as showing through agreed-upon KPIs some of the ROI items listed earlier.

Fast forward 2 years, and that CRO was able to pride itself on having one of the largest and most experienced data standard teams in the industry. Despite the primary ROI target being the efficiency gains and quality increases, that team also reached billability levels, which not only covered the cost of the entire team but also helped to become a door opener for new clients, resulting in previously unimaginable and novel revenue streams.

Summarizing the ROI Argument for CDM

From a high-level point of view, it comes down to the fact of switching the perception of CDM in your respective company, from being solely a costly commodity to a differentiating and value-generating core department.

The internal discussions should transition to the opportunities a state-of-the-art CDM department can bring to the table for the entire company, regardless of whether the company is a service provider or pharma/biotech company. This does not mean that cost-related and efficiency-driving topics should not be discussed. Absolutely they should! However, they should be part of the full CDM ROI discussion and not the sole target.

As mentioned earlier, anybody working in a CDM team, from the individual contributor who is just starting a career in CDM, to the experienced veteran in senior leadership, has to have a constant desire to show and increase the value of this pivotal department. There is a reason why we are not doing paper CRFs anymore!

Here is a list of possible value-adding CDM opportunities to start discussing in your respective team and company to start changing the narrative and show proactivity:

- Examine any manual process step and check for options to automate
- New technologies that can reduce process steps and centralize data
- Look at all touch points and handovers with other functional areas
- Review all major and critical quality issues of the last 24 months and find innovative ways to ensure they won't repeat. Did the implemented CAPAs hold up?
- For service providers – find new value driving revenue opportunities

How to Measure and Present Success for a CDM Department

Now that we have established the foundations by establishing the right culture first and understanding how to spearhead investment in CDM toward a meaningful ROI in your respective company, let's take the final step toward CDS advocacy.

As the subtitle of this paragraph already suggests, CDM professionals who expand the footprint into data science will have to constantly measure progress and present on either the success of the steps taken toward data science or take the necessary actions to turn failing initiatives into positive ones.

What does this mean and what needs to be measured and presented?

Remember, many of the intricacies of CDM will remain a nebulous area for most of your colleagues in other functions around you. Having oversight through KPIs and the ability to visualize (ideally through standardized dashboards) will allow you to address and inform any internal or external audiences when needed.

Let's look at a few examples:

Example 1: Your colleagues in Clinical Operations need (clinical) data to monitor site performance.

One example of data science going beyond the traditional CDM tasks is to take on the role of providing data, tools, dashboards, and part of the narrative when it comes to enabling Clinical Operations to perform the task of site oversight. Identifying underperforming, suspicious, insufficiently trained, over/under-reporting, quality concerning, and non-complaint sites is part of Clinical Operation' remit; however, CDM has the tools and data to *measure* and guide this oversight.

Example 2: Regular conference attendance and active involvement in industry-leading discussions by all levels of staff.

Coming to the "presenting" part of CDM's success, it is very helpful to have a comparator. What is the objective benchmark for all those measurements we are talking about? Being able to quote and refer to industry's "voice" in company internal meetings is very helpful. It can become the main argument for crucial investments, assignment of tasks, or understanding what success actually looks like. This will not happen overnight, but this should not deter the effort of rewarding motivated staff to attend and present at industry events and, on the same token, strive to be a role model leader who engages in leadership events as well.

The obvious benefit of having these industry events in your back pocket is the resulting ability to take subjectivity out of your argumentation strategy and be able to build your case on the objective regulatory and industry's best practices framework.

Example 3: CRO – Pharma/Biotech (i.e. sponsor) interactions.

Regardless of which side of the discussion you represent in your CDM role, having a broad and diverse background with a solid understanding of CDS's best practices and regulatory framework will increase your chances of being an effective CDM leader dramatically.

Either by being clearly able to articulate your service needs from a sponsor perspective and to provide the required oversight of the CRO, or by being able to guide sponsor companies effectively from a CRO perspective.

Let's get even more concrete.

Being part of a CDM team that aims to extract maximum value out of clinical data must not only cover the basic items but also drive toward and *advocate* for showing the additional value that can be gained.

A few of the basic and decades-old items are:

- Number of new, open, closed, and reissued queries
- Missing page reports
- Pages with missing flags (e.g., SDV, signed) or ready-to-freeze/lock
- Updates on progress of reconciliation activities and medical coding
- Perform required database updates when needed

Yes, these are part of the CDM job; however, the true value comes with the move toward CDS and leading the way for:

- Prevention of data-related issues rather than post hoc fixing them
- Early detection of data anomalies
- Cross-functional alignment on execution of data integrity strategies
- Getting closer and closer to the true source of the data
- Ensure robust data even in more complex settings such as:
  - Adaptive clinical trials
  - Basket or umbrella studies
  - Novel therapeutic approaches which require unique data collection and review methodologies
- Supporting the updated regulatory framework of risk-based approaches and focusing on critical-to-success factors

The latter list is needed for most studies, and companies will find ways to address these needs. However, if this void is not filled by CDS Advocates and Leaders, it will be filled by other functions who in many cases do not have the affinity with, and dare I say "feeling" for, clinical data. This again is unfortunately not a hypothetical statement, as I do come across too many companies, where the complexity of these items is underestimated and the pseudo-solutions insufficient.

The obvious and already proven win-win scenario is for CDM to fill this void. The win for CDM lies within the fact of the continuous expansion of our profession, as we have been doing it for decades now in the face of technological advances and the changing regulatory requirements.

The more important win though is for our industry as a whole. CDM, using its talent, background, experience, and passion for data-driven approaches, is the key to unlocking the pathway toward the ultimate goal of clinical research: to bring new and innovative lifesaving and quality-of-life-improving medicines to *more* patients *quicker*.

How do we measure success and can prove the added value?

Execution of any clinical study is always, without exception, a bumpy ride. Some bumps can be so critical and result in derailing an entire study, putting patient lives at risk, or be the reason for not getting marketing approval by regulatory agencies.

Therefore, it is very valuable to measure the reduction of bumps and the complete avoidance of the truly critical ones.

To ensure a smoother ride, a successful CDM department with state-of-the-art CDS processes should do the following:

- Rigorously track and present status and trends of critical-to-success factors and the underlying data, as well as suggesting and implementing remediation measures for identified risks
- Review of protocol designs to ensure that the to-be-collected data is sufficient and relevant to support the main goals of the study, as well as optimizing the collection processes and tools
- Lead the cross-functional team in striving toward a unified and timely data review effort, to avoid a bolus of unreviewed data
- Lead the discussion and become the key decision maker for any technology used to collect, review, or touch clinical data in any way
- Establish a clear communication plan and escalation path with all relevant parties, for example, CRO, Sponsor, third-party data provider, technology providers

This is not an exhaustive list; however, it should provide enough references on how to approach the task of Data Science implementation and execution. Looking at the relevant calls for action of this list, we see "Track", "Review", "Optimize", "Lead", "Key Decision Maker", and "Clear communication plan", as a result, the overall direction to take and mindset to have should be clearer now.

The tangible and measurable results, which should be presented at department meetings, town hall meetings, and when possible, at executive leadership meetings, are:

- Reduction of database unlocks.
- Reduction of CDM-related protocol amendments.
- Reduction of clinical-data-related findings in audits.
- Increase in data review efficiency linked to reduction of duplications. This can be shown by analyzing a reduction in issued queries, site and CRA feedback, as well as the reduced time to database lock or other key milestones.

- Reduction of protocol deviations, because of early detection.
- Reduction of critical escalations, because of the established communication plans, which will ensure that daily items get addressed at the lowest possible level.

Again, this list is easily extendable, when the right culture, processes, and management support are in place.

Over time some more subtle benefits will emerge as well. Colleagues from other functions and study team members from other companies will start trusting CDM. Adding regular active industry attendances, that is, representing your company at those events by leading a discussion topic, preparing a poster for an exhibit, presenting a case study on a panel, or volunteering for a committee will further cement your department's positive perception.

To be clear, these external engagements are and should not be limited just to senor leaders in the CDM department. There are ample opportunities to get actively involved in CDM-related industry events for all levels. You do not have to be 10+ year CDM veteran to share your experience on a topic you feel passionate about.

Lastly, your and the CDM department's reputation and positive trajectory will have to exhibit a constant desire toward further improvement and adjustment to keep up with industry trends and the changing demand from a regulatory and technological point of view. There is no standstill in CDM and in our industry. Not innovating, not adjusting, or unwillingness to step out of comfort zones is equivalent to starting the erosion of CDM and its value in any environment.

This is one of the many fascinating aspects of being a CDM professional and developing a desire to push the envelope toward CDS Advocacy.

Summary

Using the background of more traditional CDM approaches, we have now seen how to use this basis as a foundation for starting the journey toward CDS. Even though it might seem to be a CDM self-promoting push to put our profession at the helm of the clinical data discussions, the tangible examples shared in this chapter should show the true value for the respective company enjoying the benefits of an innovative and motivated CDM team.

It is my hope that this chapter will have sparked your desire and triggered ideas for you directly or for your respective department to start, continue, or expand your journey toward CDM excellence and data science advocacy.

In this chapter on overall CDM value creation, we looked at ROI, measurement of success, and the required culture in more general terms. I now look forward to reflecting on my own professional evolution from a clueless programmer who stumbled into CDM by accident 30+ years ago and is now making a living from being an executive leader in one of the top Biometrics companies in the industry.

Let's get personal!

9

From Programmer to Executive – A Personal Story

We have reached the final chapter, and I want to thank you, dear reader, for the time you have already dedicated to getting to this point. Together we have explored the unique opportunity that CDM professionals have at their fingertips, to make a difference for patients, clinical research in general, and the institutions we work for.

In this last part of the book, I now feel comfortable sharing my personal story with you. The intent is to have it serve you as a real-life example and hopefully inspire and motivate you to either take the first steps now in your career toward more influential assignments or push farther from where you currently are on your own professional trajectory.

Among other areas, we will touch on the importance of having mentors, identify signs that suggest changing your current work environment, and learn how to build meaningful professional networks. Similar to the previous chapters, I will also be providing real-life examples to illustrate more tangibly a given topic.

The main goal of this chapter is to show you the numerous opportunities this industry holds for our profession and to encourage you to give it a try for yourself to push for your maximum potential.

To do so, we will look at:

- The mentor
- The power of networking
- Leadership and legacy

The Mentor

Another Sunday afternoon sitting at Washington Dulles Airport waiting for the boarding process for the third transatlantic flight I am taking this year, and we are only in spring. This 12-day trip includes several client meetings,

DOI: 10.1201/9781003648314-9

as well as a speaking slot as session chair at SCDM on topics related to RBQM and AI. The highlight of this trip, however, is a planned Gala Dinner organized by the Founder and CEO of the company I joined a few months earlier, to announce my official start as their new President.

Client meetings? Public speaking at prestigious industry forums? President of a company? How did all of that happen?

It feels like yesterday, well not really "yesterday" as we are talking 30+ years, but the memories are still vivid of me struggling, and sometimes failing, to get passing grades in my English classes, or the stomachache before a teleconference with our US colleagues, because of the fear of not understanding what they say, or even worse . . . maybe having to speak.

I want to get closer to answer the question of which factors, circumstances, decisions, people, or percentage of luck did, in combination, provide the opportunity to open the doors for me to go from a mediocre, at best, CDM Programmer to Company Executive.

So let us start at the beginning. I was born in the early 1970s in the heart of the industrial coalmining region of Germany, The Ruhrgebiet, and raised in a blue-collar environment.

The one truly valuable distinguishing factor early on though, which is worthwhile pointing out, was the fact that due to my mother being from Spain – Catalonia to be more specific – I was raised bilingual.

In kindergarten and school, and with my father and German grandparents, I only spoke German, and with my mother exclusively Catalan and adding Spanish to the mix later on. This resulted in me being able to speak these three languages rather fluently from a very early age. The true value of this gift became obvious to me much later in life.

We can quickly skip the 13 years I spent in the German school system, as they were unremarkable. Just a regular kid, being the youngest in my classes in all of the 13 years, due to an early start in kindergarten, and therefore often picked on by older classmates. In my recollection of those events, it did not seem to bother me too much and just might have fostered the basis of being able to stand on my own feet and not becoming discouraged or embarrassed easily when facing adversity.

All throughout the scholastic journey my interests in mathematical and scientific-oriented classes grew. This then resulted in me selecting Mathematics, Physics, Philosophy, and Sports as the four focus areas of my final school years and allowed me to finish my "Abitur" (the German "Gymnasium" [Highschool] final exams) in 1990, with a 2.1 grade average on a scale from 1 = Highest possible, to 6 = Insufficient. A result which did not represent anything outstanding, but good enough to open doors for starting a secondary education or college degrees.

We are now approaching possibly the first pivotal moment of my career. An early example of taking a step toward an unknown future and getting out of a relatively cozy environment, paired with an element of luck.

The relatively limited options at hand for me at that time were to continue my secondary education at a traditional university close by and stay home, or to opt for a combined study and work environment which were offered by some of the larger corporations in Germany.

Even at this early age, I was just approaching my 19th birthday, I had a sense that hands-on work experience, paired with continuous education and pursuing a degree, was more valuable than just studying for another 4+ years and then trying to enter the workforce at 24+.

Therefore, I applied for two of these programs. One at Bayer in Leverkusen, for a Programming role with an attached degree in the equivalent of what is known today as computer science, and the other one at Hoechst in Frankfurt, as Lab Physicist, with a degree in Physics.

Either one of these options would require me to leave my home, friends, and known environment for either Leverkusen or Frankfurt.

Early summer of 1990 I received the rejection from Bayer but got an invitation to Frankfurt to take an entry exam and interview for the Lab Physicists position at Hoechst. I have to admit that at this stage I had not a real good understanding of what this role would entail, but "Lab" sounded scientific, and "Physicist" sounded close enough to the areas of interest that I had in school. With the prospect of being able to eventually get a college degree, get hands-on work experience, and earn some money, I accepted the invitation and went the 220 km (≈135 miles) to Frankfurt to take the entry exam.

I recall the sleepless night before the exam day, and the walk to the exam place on the Hoechst campus in my cheap off-the-shelve suit, which I had just bought a few days earlier aiming for a slightly more professional look. The exam turned out to be more mathematical-oriented than expected and in the following interview, when discussing the results, I was told that I had scored relatively high in the mathematical sections and less well in the physics areas, which opened the door for a different pathway at Hoechst – The "Industry Computer Scientist".

As a quick reminder for you, this was 1990. Personal computers (PCs) were just emerging, and most private households did not own a PC. Companies in general were in transition mode from typewriters and manual processes to open up more tech-driven information centers.

At the time, I did not realize the lucky break I just had, thanks to the test results and not being discarded for the Lab Physicist role but considered for the Industry Computer Scientist Role.

I did accept the role and had now a few months to prepare my permanent move away from home to Frankfurt and start my pursuit of a Computer Scientist and Mathematics degree, as well as the hands-on work opportunities offered by the company.

I am now excited to share with you one of the weirdest twists and lucky coincidences that enabled my career in clinical research and introduce you to one of my first mentors – Oscar Vanderbeke, Head of the Biometrics Department at Hoechst in the early 1990s.

The backstory is the following. My parallel tracks of working at Hoechst and studying in the company's integrated college meant that students like me would be randomly assigned to a department in need of computer science resources for an 8-month long deployment, while continuing all study assignments.

My first two assignments had been initially inside of a chemistry laboratory, writing Quick Basic Code to control experimental machinery, whereas the second assignment was part of the agricultural branch of Hoechst and program dBase – databases for collection and management of data originating from experimental pesticides, fungicides, and herbicides tested on company-owned farms.

The third and final assignment was the most important one, as it typically meant that after successful completion of your college degree, you would remain in that department for your full-time occupation after graduation. For that final assignment, I had been preselected to join again the same chemistry laboratory I had spent my first 8 months at, because at that time programmers with Quick Basik knowledge were rare.

However, destiny, possibly luck, and most importantly Mister Oscar Vanderbeke intervened. At the time, I did not know Oscar, and he did not know me; however, we both shared a very unusual passion – Prime Numbers, and the mathematical mysteries and oddities related to them.

Just a few weeks before the final assignment needed to be confirmed, I had a breakthrough in my prime number explorations and had found a record-breaking prime number formula, representing the longest chain of prime numbers in a row, created by an exponential function. Concretely, it was $f(X) = 4^X + 4503$, for which for all $f(X)$ are prime for $X = 1, 2, 3, \ldots, 14$.

This fact was picked up by a local newspaper; the internal *Hoechst Magazine* published an article (see Figure 9.1) on this, and this was included in a math book dedicated to mathematical mysteries.

Oscar had seen the article in the company's magazine and decided to invite me for an informal chat in his office in Hoechst's clinical research facility.

As you can imagine, at first, I was quite nervous to sit down with one of the company's executives; however, Oscar had such a warm, open, and welcoming approach that I felt at ease quickly. The result of this conversation was that he was looking for some help with his own prime number curiosities, which I happily provided over the next days in my limited spare time.

Two weeks before starting my third and last company work assignment at the chemistry laboratory, I was called into the dean's office and asked if I were rather interested in starting a position as SAS-Programmer in the clinical research facility, as Oscar Vanderbeke had reached out to see, if I could become part of his team. The twists of destiny to get to this point were unbelievable. The odds of finding a record breaking formula at the right time, and this news being noticed by the Head of a Biometrics Department, who also happened to share the same passion, must have been astronomically low. But this perfect star alignment was the start of my clinical research carer.

I spent the next 8 months during my final work assignment as part of the clinical research team and learned SAS as a new programming language, and yes, Oscar and I spent an occasional coffee break together talking about

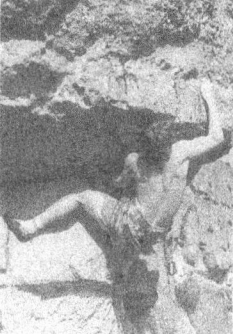

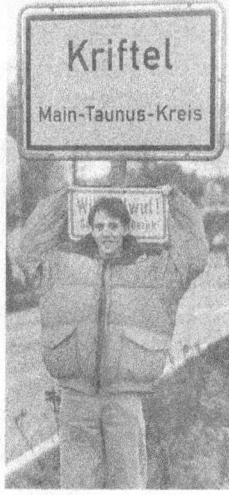

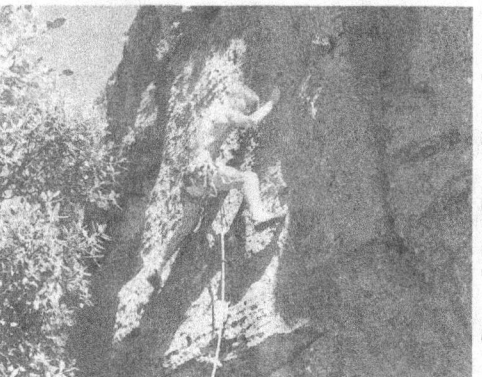

Bilder links und unten: Michael Gödde ist nicht nur „Zahlen-Fan" und Rekordbrecher beim Finden von Primzahlen, sondern auch begeisterter Freeclimber – eine waghalsige Angelegenheit, wie unsere Fotos zeigen. Hier sehen wir ihn „in action" beim Erklettern des „La Masura" in der Nähe von Tarragona in Spanien.

Tagtäglich versuchen viele Menschen, alte Rekorde zu überbieten. Sei es beim Essen von Negerküssen oder nur beim längsten Tauchgang in der heimischen Badewanne! Man findet aber auch Leute, die ihr Glück auf mathematischem Gebiet suchen. Sie bilden allerdings eine verschwindend kleine Minderheit. Einer von ihnen ist Michael Gödde, ein 20jähriger Industrieinformatiker im zweiten Lehrjahr bei Hoechst. Er fühlt sich zu Zahlen hingezogen wie andere zu Briefmarken oder Münzen.

Was ist denn so besonders an Zahlen? Eigentlich nichts, aber es gibt da eine Familie von Zahlen, die schon viele Mathematiker beschäftigt hat und immer noch beschäftigt: die Primzahlen! Was sind denn das für Zahlen, wird sich manch einer fragen. Michael erklärt es uns: „Primzahlen sind Zahlen, die genau zwei Teiler haben, zum Beispiel die 2, 3, 5, 7, 11, 13. Die Mathematiker sind auf der Suche nach immer größeren Primzahlen und nach Möglichkeiten, diese irgendwie bestimmen zu können."

Durch Zufall entdeckte Michael in einem Buch eine Exponentialgleichung der Form $y = ax^n + h$, die für $n = 1, \ldots, 6$ Primzahlen erzeugt. Der Autor stellte diese Formel als einzigartig hin. Das weckte erst recht Michaels Interesse, so daß er einen großen Teil seiner Freizeit damit verbrachte, weitere Formeln zu finden, die noch mehr Primzahlen liefern. Und wie es halt so ist im richtigen Leben, er fand tatsächlich eine Formel, die mehr als sechs Primzahlen lieferte! Die festen Parameter a, x und b wurden durch gezieltes Probieren gesucht. Von einem Mathematiker erhielt er den Hinweis, daß jede Primzahl sich durch $6 \times \pm 1$ darstellen läßt.

„Die kleineren Primzahlen konnte ich noch per Hand überprüfen, aber dann mußte doch der Rechner ran", erklärt mir Michael. Seine zuletzt gefundene Gleichung erzeugt 14 Primzahlen für alle $n = 1, \ldots, 14$ und überbietet damit die Gleichung im Buch um mehr als das Doppelte. Daraufhin nahm er Kontakt mit dem Autor auf, der begeistert war über die Entdeckung und ihm eine Erwähnung in der Neuauflage versprach!

Bei den Exponentialgleichungen glaubt Michael an einem Punkt angekommen zu sein, an dem es nicht weitergeht, denn es tut sich nichts mehr auf dem Rechner. Deshalb hat er als nächstes Ziel vor, das Polynom von Euler $y = x^2 + x + 41$, das sogar 40 Primzahlen liefert, zu übertrumpfen.

Michael hat aber noch ganz andere Hobbys, die mit diesem Spleen nichts gemein haben: Er ist begeisterter Freeclimber, wie man den Bildern ansehen kann. Und da soll noch einer behaupten, Mathematiker wären Stubenhocker…

Die Frage, ob er sich nach seiner Ausbildung hauptsächlich der Primzahlsuche widmen wird, dementiert er: Er will auch in Zukunft bei Hoechst bleiben, wenn möglich bei Hoechst Ibérica, denn er ist Halbspanier!

Frank Schönberg

FIGURE 9.1
Hoechst Magazine Article.

prime numbers. After my graduation, I was able to fill a full-time position in clinical research as a Statistical Programmer 1 and start my actual career in clinical research. Until his eventual retirement in the mid-1990s, Oscar continued to be very generous with his time and shared valuable insights from his decade-long career with me. Despite the generational gap between us and the obvious gap in level, title, and experience, I felt empowered and allowed to make mistakes to learn.

Why am I sharing this with you? In my mind, I think that Oscar exhibited so many key characteristics of an ideal mentor, which will help you to either become a mentor yourself, or, if you are lucky enough, become a mentee, of somebody like Oscar.

Looking at these characteristics, concretely I mean the following:

- Willing to take a risk with somebody who is junior and inexperienced.
- Altruistic, in the sense that the mentor's main intent is to just help somebody else by passing on his/her knowledge, without serving any self-interests.
- Open to work with people from different generations, backgrounds, or educational levels.
- Ability to identify hidden talents or assets within people that can be unlocked through targeted coaching.
- Comfortable breaking through corporate siloes, and hierarchical or political structures of companies.

I think that Oscar's influence at the very early stages of my career, as well as the coincidence of our shared passion for prime numbers, and the lucky timing of me making a headline around this topic right when the last work assignments had to be made are just a few components of sometimes the stars aligning. These are the moments when decisions need to be made, by the mentor and the mentee, to move ahead and to seize the opportunity. I can say with confidence that without the courage from both ends, it is very likely that I would have had a career as Programmer in that chemistry laboratory, without even knowing that an industry in clinical research even existed.

Over the next years in my career, I enjoyed my existence as a Programmer in the clinical research center of Hoechst and started building and expanding my technical skills around Programming, basic CDM tasks, the early industry discussions around data standards, and cross-functional discussions with Clinical Operations and other departments. I was on the standard professional path of spending my entire working life at this company and in this same role until retiring as Senior Principal Programmer, or equivalent level, at the end.

There was no realistic prospect toward any sort of managerial or higher-level roles for people in my position, because of the very restricted and (over-) regulated processes in German companies at that time.

Looking back at that period of my career, I think the possibly surprising, sad, or scary part of it was that I had accepted that fact and was overall okay with the prospects I had.

With this background in mind, I will introduce you now to the most significant and influential mentor throughout my professional career – Hugh Donovan. The person who made me find, recognize, and develop capabilities and talents I did not even know I possessed. The person who, on the one hand, I could count on to back me up publicly and who, on the other hand, would call me out in private settings with brutal honesty and directness. The person that showed me that "good" is never "good enough" and that the strive for excellence is a never-ending journey. And lastly, the person who helped me to build the courage and confidence to be my authentic true self in any setting.

In the mid- to late 1990s Hoechst went through several transformations due to Merger and Acquisition (M&A) activities. In short succession Hoechst became Hoechst Roussel and then Hoechst Marion Roussel (HMR), after the respective mergers with Roussel Uclaf and with Marion Merrell Dow.

In 1999, the Hoechst name got eliminated from the Pharma sector completely, when HMR merged with Rhône-Poulenc to not become HMRRP (maybe a good decision), but a fresh "new" company – Aventis.

In those years, my first mentor, Oscar, had retired and together with many of my local programming colleagues, we had to get used to a much more global environment, with new colleagues from France, England, and most significantly with our counterparts in the newly established Headquarters in Bridgewater, New Jersey, USA.

The switch from a 99+% German work environment to English was particularly hard for me, as my 9 years of struggles through my English classes in school were not sufficient to give me the confidence to be able to participate actively and meaningfully in any meetings conducted in English.

At that time, Hugh Donovan was our US-based VP of the global Biometrics department. He would come to visit the Frankfurt office a few times a year and hold departmental town hall meetings with all local staff, followed by a few smaller group meetings and a few one-on-ones with select individuals.

At the beginning, these town hall meetings were nerve-wracking for me, as our entire department of about 50 people would be attending to listen to Hugh's latest announcements, followed by a Q&A block.

However, after having had the chance to experience Hugh in a couple of these meetings and encouraged by the earlier experiences with senior leadership through my interactions with Oscar, I did volunteer to present two small topics at the upcoming townhall meeting. One was related to my support role as a CDM SAS Programmer for a cardiovascular mega trial, and the other topic was to share with Hugh that people in Frankfurt had some concerns around our work environment in Germany after all those mergers.

In the days leading up to the meeting I prepared some slides, which needed to be placed manually on an overhead projector to see the image on the wall. I distinctly recall how with slightly shaky and sweaty hands I was trying to place the slides on the projector the right way up and say the words I had rehearsed so many times before.

Now asking again, why do I share these details with you? – Many reasons.

Stepping Out of Your Comfort Zone

Let me start by pointing out that this must have been the first example in my career of having stepped out of my comfort zone, without an obvious need of having been forced to do so. Remember, I did volunteer to do this!

Why? I can assure you it was definitely not to somehow look for recognition or distinguish myself, but the inner voice that we all have that was telling me that there were things that needed to be said, and Hugh needed to hear them.

Leadership Style

In Hugh's earlier meetings, I had observed how respectfully he treated people even if he disagreed with them, how his seniority and title did not seem to matter, and his focus to strive to understand the root cause of any possible issue. I would likely not have found the courage to volunteer to present and speak my mind using subpar English, if Hugh had not had the leadership style, which he exhibited in every word he said and every action he took. I felt and ultimately knew that he did value people, regardless of their level and positions in the company, to just speak their mind.

This is something so fundamental when trying to foster a culture based on trust and to build and grow a global department. This is just one of so many characteristics that I learned from Hugh firsthand and have been trying to emulate in my later career stages.

Becoming a Mentor/Mentee

Oscar or Hugh never said to me: "Hello Michael, I think I should be your mentor", and I had never asked to be mentored. The uniqueness of these two leaders, differentiating them from the average leader, was that their actions, aura, words, selflessness, and direct feedback encouraged people, who were open for advice and ready to embrace change, even if uncomfortable, to gravitate naturally toward them. You do not become a mentor by announcing it, but by exhibiting constant exemplary behavior in the form of respecting every individual surrounding you and allow for every opinion to have a chance to be heard. In addition, a basis of trust needs to be formed by authenticity and a rigorous follow-up on actions to the words you say.

After this townhall meeting, I had my first one-on-one meeting with Hugh. He told me that he was very interested in the possible data issues I had found for the cardiovascular mega study and that he valued the fact that I had brought some of the departmental sentiments to his attention. I felt heard! Even though I am sure he did not agree with some of my statements, which came through as he stated his points of view, I was just relieved that somebody senior had listened.

After this initial meeting, our one-on-one meetings became more regular during his visits to Frankfurt, and I gained more confidence in my English skills speaking with Hugh and through more interactions with other US counterparts.

As I had pointed out earlier in the characteristics of mentors taking risks and giving people opportunities, this was exactly what Hugh did for me. Despite being just an average programmer, at best, and having more experienced people around me, I did find myself more and more involved in task-forces focused on departmental activities around SOPs and Data Standards and on sharing best practices with global teams.

It culminated with Hugh putting the gears in motion to offer me eventually a relocation from Frankfurt, Germany, to Bridgewater, NJ, to join his global team of Project Data Managers (PDMs) in the global headquarters. Even though it took me 2 years to eventually accept his offer, he never gave up on the idea to have me, this outspoken, unfiltered (at least back then), half-German, half Spanish guy join his handpicked mix of global PDMs he had formed.

The same way a decade earlier, Oscar took a gamble with me, by bringing a Quick Basic Programmer into clinical research; it is solely thanks to Hugh that in September of 2001 my family moved to Bridgewater, and I did my first significant and meaningful career step, by becoming a PDM with global project responsibilities.

Hugh's and my intertwined journey continued for a few more years at that company and little did we know then that our professional paths would cross again a decade later.

Moving on from the importance of allowing the right mentors into your life, graciously accepting the role of mentee, starting to put the puzzle pieces together to eventually strive for opportunities to pay back and mentor people yourself, and passing on the legacy from those who came before us.

The Power of Networking

I had the privilege to lead some academy programs for companies I worked for, giving me the opportunity to engage with university students. In these discussions I get asked often about key factors for building a successful career. The people inquiring about this seem to expect answers involving higher level degrees or other forms of continuous education. Yes, having a solid academic background is definitely part of a promising foundation;

however, what I usually tell these students, or other people in early stages of their career, is that building an international and interdisciplinary network is another important piece of the puzzle.

Through more modern and affordable means of transportation the world has become smaller. I am convinced that my passion, borderline obsession, for exploring every possible corner of the world and experiencing new cultures, being confronted with new norms, and having to find the delicate balance between respectfully embracing the unknown surroundings while still carrying one's identity are the best life lessons a person can get.

Thus, my recommendations for those audiences typically include the encouragement to travel, to explore, to ask questions, to widen horizons, to engage with other cultures, and to be proud of one's heritage and origin, while remaining always open to learn and adapt from these experiences.

Asking the "why" question again. We are looking at career pathways from Programmer, or any other individual contributor role, to executive-level roles.

I do immensely respect those individuals who have found their passion in a non-managerial and less strategic-oriented work assignment, because after many years of experience in a dedicated role, many become an SME for a given area. These people are tremendously valuable in any organization.

However, if from the beginning of your career or realizing over time that the aim for you is to take on more strategic and senior roles, which often involve global accountabilities, an understanding of the nuanced and sometime less-nuanced differences of cultures in your team is pivotal to success.

Picking up on my own journey in the early 2000s, after moving with my family from Germany to the US, my industry network was still rather limited, despite a good amount of international travel.

In my role as PDM one main reason for travel was Investigator Meetings, where PDMs would present the CDM portion of a given clinical study together with the other functional representatives. Other occasions for travel were meetings with the CDM service providers we were using. I was happy in my role as I was getting more comfortable with my English skills which allowed me to become more vocal on CDM-related items and continued to benefit from Hugh's helpful guidance and occasional push.

It is only fair at this point in time to also mention the influence Abdelhak Oualim, another "Hugh-Alumni" and my direct Manager, had on me with his focus on excellence in delivery for all CDM tasks.

To put things into perspective, I was about 12–13 years into my career and did not really have an ambition to go for any managerial role, as I did not see it suited with my more technical background and the absence of an advanced degree.

Things would have likely continued like this for many more years, possibly until the end of my career, if it weren't for some significant events in the early 2000s and Hugh's gracious support and interventions.

In 2004, after 3 years in the US, I had built a solid reputation as a PDM, had been promoted to Senior PDM, and had led CDM activities for two of our company's top pipeline candidates toward submission.

The first key event, which still influences my career today, was Hugh opening the opportunity for me (once again) to attend the SCDM annual conference in Toronto. I had heard about SCDM from a distance due to Hugh's role as Chair in 2001, and some of our leadership attending previous conferences, but did not really know what to expect. The thought of having to be co-presenting in two sessions did make me nervous.

I will spare you the unflattering details of my state of mind the night before my presentations and the hours and minutes leading up to the actual events. However, in the end, like with so many things in life, it turned out that the actual event, the act of speaking in a non-native language, with a heavy foreign accent, and a slightly shaky voice, which likely only I felt, was not as bad as the angst I had built up in my head.

I am not ashamed at all of sharing these, almost intimate, details with you, because I want to believe that you either went through a similar experience already in your career and do understand, or you will eventually face a similar situation and hopefully be comforted that we all sweat bullets at some point in time.

More important, though, than just logging my first two official "publications" for my CV was the energy I felt at SCDM. There was a NETWORK of people from all sorts of different companies, talking openly about the same issues and possible solutions, that I had faced myself in the last 10+ years. This was also the time in CDM and the industry with the quite divisive topic of Paper versus EDC.

For the first time in my career, it felt that handing out business cards and receiving some in return actually made sense. LinkedIn and QR codes were not born yet.

Thus, the first key item in 2004 was my eye-opening experience at the first industry event I attended and realizing that the CDM world went way beyond my company's horizon I had had until then. There was a broader vision and mission for CDM professionals out there, rather than just locking databases, and there was a network of people out there influencing progress in the industry. That had left an impression on me.

Two decades later a small sample of the conference badges I collected looks like this (Figure 9.2).

The second significant event in that period, which created a chain reaction, was a hostile takeover by another company. Up to that point, I was no stranger to mergers and companies coming together, but this one was different in nature.

With this takeover, new and very important learnings for me were around the corner.

In the early days, going through the normal restructuring that was to be expected, I got accepted by the new CDM leadership to take on the role of Global Therapeutic Area Head for Oncology and Neurology. This was the first managerial role in my career and entailed the oversight of a combined team of about 40 people in the US and Europe.

Hugh had been instrumental at convincing me that I was ready for this role and then pushing it through the necessary approval steps.

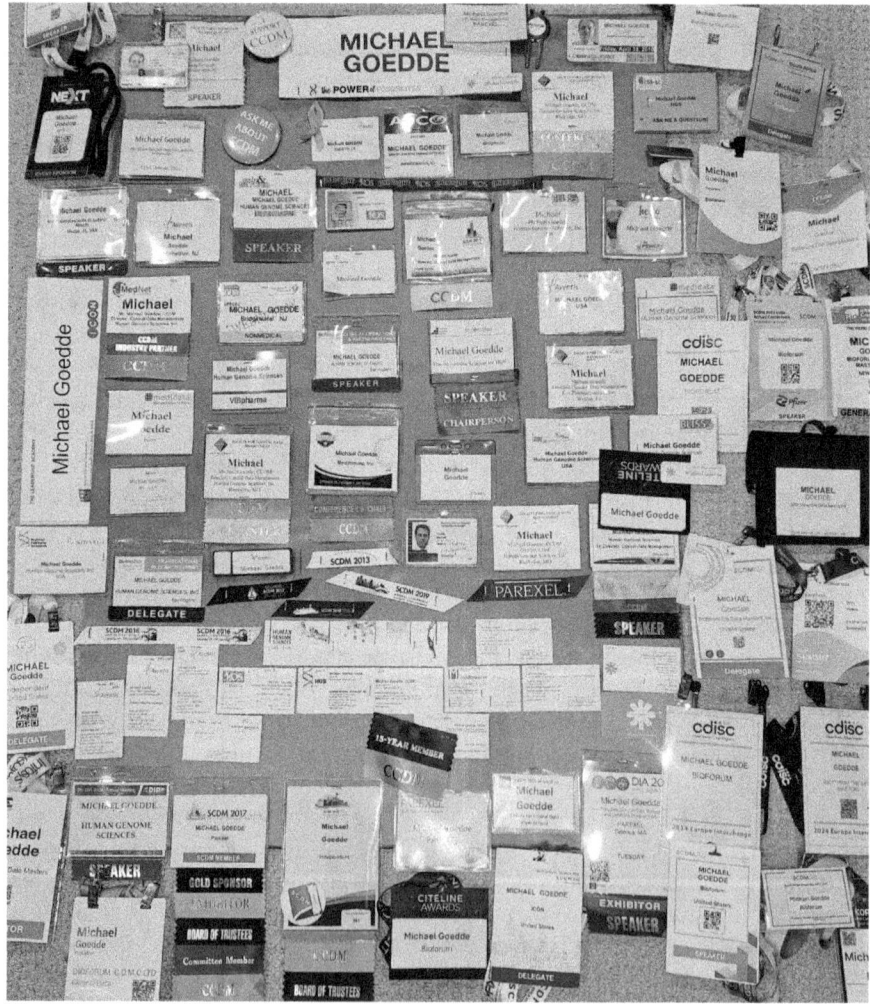

FIGURE 9.2
Sample of conference badges and other network events.

To my dismay, shortly thereafter Hugh was made redundant, exited the company, and the Biometrics department with CDM moved to new leadership.

Even though on paper it appeared to be a significant step moving from Senior PDM to the level of Associate Director in the aforementioned role, the reality turned out to be completely different.

For the first time I was exposed to a new company culture that felt very different to what I had experienced previously. CDM continued to be a big department, but the standing and internal reputation seemed to be diminished and in the shadow of the Clinical Department.

I quickly realized that outspoken CDM representatives, like me and many of my previous colleagues, were a new experience for the newly formed teams.

CDM as a function was seen as purely operational and a commodity, rather than a strategic area of expertise that is accountable for the end-to-end data flow toward overall quality.

This mismatch culminated in one of the most memorable comments, yet hurtful in the moment, I have received in my professional career, coming from a superior.

After an intense discussion with the medical directors and clinical operations representatives on data standards for the therapeutic areas I was accountable for, where I was trying to explain the importance of adherence to such standards, I was told "Michael, when a clinical person is in the room, CDM shuts up!"

That was, at the same time, the beginning of the end for me at that company, as well as the exciting start of something new.

Eight months later I took the right, yet painful, decision to quit my job after 15 years at that company.

I am sharing this with you, as the valuable lesson I can pass on with this example is that despite the disappointment of having to leave the company that I valued so much, that had given me my education and allowed me to grow in my early years; there can come the point when you must move on.

This point is reached when despite one's best efforts a change will not be possible, and the walls become unsurmountable.

At this point in my career my network was still rather limited, and I had to rely on previous colleagues or the few external contacts I had.

Fast forwarding the next 2 years, I became Head of CDM at a Biotech company in Florida under the leadership of one of my previous colleagues.

It was only a short engagement in Florida, as that company also got bought by a larger pharma company.

The two memorable episodes I recall from my time in Florida were the audit in Moscow, which I already shared in detail in Chapter 2 as well as one particular budget discussion I had with my superior.

The CDM department was due to submit our annual budget needs for CDM in terms of technology expansions. Even though we were not too happy with our current technology solutions, as they seemed outdated and required a lot of manual work, we were just scraping by due to the phenomenal team we had been able to form in that short period of time.

In the meeting itself, my superior told me that he had calculated a total investment budget of about $50k for the year to address some minor patches and upgrades, whereas on my piece of paper I had a number of $600k to go with a major overhaul of our technology landscape.

Pivotal moment coming up! My superior had mentioned his $50k first and explained his reasoning. He did not know what I had on my piece of paper.

Do I take the possibly easier way and just agree with his suggestion, or do I risk being perceived as out of touch with reality with a 12-fold higher number?

In this case it was a rather easy decision from my end, as I knew that my superior values my honest opinion, he absolutely exhibited in all his actions the willingness to listen, and we both understood the value of transparency.

After an initial laugh, as he thought I was joking when I mentioned my number, he quickly saw the strategic benefits of the case presented, adjusted his point of view, and, most importantly, had the boldness and determination to bring the $600k proposal to executive leadership. He took the risk!

The new CDM budget proposal was presented, with the outcome of getting an allocation of $600k + $X, if needed, as the company did understand the value of Clinical Data and that it was not an area for cheap corner cutting or manual patch work and listened to the SMEs from each department.

I am certain that the same scenario at a company with a less open culture, more hierarchical politics, and a more self-serving leader would have resulted in a very different outcome.

After the company in Florida got bought, I moved with my family to Maryland to join another, similarly sized Biotech company as Director of CDM.

Happy to share a valuable inside with you, especially if you are at the stage in your career, when you are moving toward Director+ positions.

I learned a valuable lesson from my new Manager at Maryland Biotech.

I found myself in a new environment, where most people had never heard about me before and without the usual support network I had at previous companies, I had this nagging feeling that I had to prove myself very quickly. At that point in time, I had more than 15 years of experience in the field and thought that I had a good grip on industry's best practices.

Rather than giving myself time in the first 2–3 months to first listen to my new team of about 40 professionals, assess the situation of the department, and identify true areas of improvement, I started on the completely wrong foot. Looking back now through the lens of time and remembering some of my early comments made and actions I took, I do feel embarrassed!

To be completely open, I think that after years of riding on a wave of positive feedback, rapid career growth, and ample industry engagement, I had become overly confident that I had the perfect answer for every CDM-related problem.

It was time for me to get a kick in the shin to bring me back to reality.

My new manager was the Kicker, and I am thankful today for what he did!

At the routine 3-month check-in meeting with him, I received one of the most direct reality checks and unfiltered feedback in my career.

Going very convinced into the meeting thinking that I was about to take my first 3 months victory lab, because of the swift actions I had taken, measurable change of pace in the team, and having drafts for process improvements ready to be implemented, I did leave that meeting thinking that I was about to lose my job and that we would have to relocate again, after just 3 months in Maryland.

His feedback revealed that, on the one hand, most people did recognize the subject matter expertise that I was bringing to the table and the undeniable passion I had behind my actions. However, on the other hand, the feedback also clearly showed that people did not feel heard.

I had completely disregarded successful processes that were working well, and lastly, I might have shocked a good number of my new direct reports with my blunt and possibly clumsy approaches.

His final statement brought it home. He said, "You have led the train out of the station, and it is a beautiful train heading very likely in the right direction, but nobody is on board!"

After this meeting, which took place on a Friday afternoon, I knew that without a change in my approach and mindset, my new job would come to an end, before it had really started.

I spent the following weekend digesting the unexpected feedback. Was he right? After all, I had worked at different companies, had tons of experience, had given a decent number of industry talks, all things that were not done at my new employer. What did they know about the industry? Was this the time for me to stand my ground and double down on my approach?

Monday morning came and I had my scheduled follow-up meeting with my superior. I was happy that I had had a few days to put things in perspective and let the original negative emotions around the previous meeting settle.

The very valuable lesson I learned in those days and thanks to him for giving me that unfiltered feedback was that even though I might have been right for many of the suggested changes, it was completely useless and irrelevant, if the people having to implement and work in the new environment were not on board with it. Building trust, accepting change, and obtaining broad support take time.

After this experience in my early days at that company, my approach when taking on new teams or joining a new company in any sort of role, especially in more strategic leadership roles, changed completely. Possibly the most significant adjustment is to really listen, not only at the beginning of a new journey, but throughout the entire work relationship, to what is on people's mind. I found that in most circumstances, the best solutions come from the people close to the actual issues in a company.

I had five very rewarding and educational years at that Biotech, with lows when one of our late-stage compounds missed its target and got rejected, but also an incredible sense of accomplishment, when we had positive results for another drug, which became the first approved Lupus drug in more than 50 years.

Thanks to that success, we drew attention again from bigger players in the market and got bought shortly after the Lupus drug was approved.

As the previous 5 years had been intense, and not even counting the 6 years prior to that with two relocations up and down the US east coast, my wife and I agreed that with our two children being 9 and 11 years old at the time, it would be a good opportunity to take a break, consider a gap year, and try homeschooling as a family.

I feel it is very important to share this more private part of my career with you, because – especially in the US, where benefits such as maternity or paternity leaves are so much shorter compared to the rest of the world, and taking more than one week vacation is frowned upon at many companies – these issues go unspoken.

It is important to periodically recharge batteries and spend meaningful time with friends and loved ones. Thus, I did take off for a total of 10 months.

It turned out to be one of the best decisions I have taken in my life. I was convinced that at time of re-entry into the workforce, my existing network, industry name recognition, and diverse CV would make it relatively easy to find a suitable position.

In those 10 months, while starting the new experience of "home" schooling, we undertook a 32-day US coast to coast RV trip, spent 7 weeks with family in Spain and Germany, and to top it off, completed an 86 days around the world trip.

These things are possible in our industry and do not have to be detrimental to anyone's career.

About 8 months into my gap year, the desire to get back to work and continue my journey to shape CDM's position in the industry grew stronger.

Through my network, I had heard that another Biotech in Maryland was trying to fill a Senior Director, Head of CDM position.

The power of having an extensive network struck again, because the Head of Biometrics at that company was an ex-colleague of mine from the previous company.

This was a great opportunity as we did not have to relocate, could continue to do homeschooling, and despite having been out of work for 10 months, I continued to advance professionally.

We are entering now the stage in my career, when thanks to my network and the reputation built over time, the number and level of professional opportunities kept growing.

Before moving along my career journey, let me provide concrete examples for you on the terms of "network" and "reputation".

Starting with – *Network*:

Network within Your Company

No matter how small or large your current company is, there are always ample opportunities for CDM professionals in any role to start building meaningful and productive work relationships. Start within your own department or through volunteering for initiatives or providing insides from your own projects at cross-functional department meetings.

The focus is on using one's knowledge not only on the possibly more targeted and default area, but also to expand it beyond the SOP-defined role.

As an example, being a CDM Programmer can be a very narrow area of responsibility within a given system or a set of tasks. However, direct access to clinical study data, paired with the CDM Programming skills, can create significant value in the form of needed dashboards for the broader study team, or better review tools for the Medical Monitors.

Network Outside of Your Company

If you work at a sponsor company, there are often opportunities to engage with service providers from technology companies or CROs. These are highly skilled people working on the same projects as you. Going through good and sometimes challenging times with these counterparts can create very strong professional bonds.

Same is true in the other direction, when you are the one working on the service provider's side and have an opportunity to work with counterparts on the sponsor side.

Network Through Industry Engagements and Volunteer Work

The ability to network through industry events, while volunteering for active roles in those events, is hands down the biggest accelerator to expand your network and grow in your profession.

I am excited to share with you a list of organizations and their respective conferences, which you should consider attending or get engaged with:

- Society for Clinical Data Management (SCDM): www.scdm.org
- Association for Clinical Data Management (ACDM): www.acdmglobal. org
- Clinical Data Interchange Standards Consortium (CDISC): www. cdsic.org
- Pharmaceutical Users Software Exchange (PHUSE): https://phuse. global
- Pharmaceutical Software User Group (PharmaSUG): www.pharmasug. org
- Scope Summit: www.scopesummit.com
- Medidata Next and Veeva Summit: www.medidata.com and www. veeva.com (under events)

As shared earlier with you, my first industry conference, SCDM 2004 in Toronto, was truly eye-opening and the dozens of subsequent events I attended in the last two decades since Toronto were without doubt the main catalyst in my career. I will be forever thankful to SCDM and the events organized by this non-profit organization and how they have helped so many professionals to learn how to lead by example in any CDM role, within their respective companies.

Moving on to – *Reputation*

There are tens of thousands of CDM professionals globally working at sponsor companies, academia, CROs, and technology companies. Despite this seemingly large number, there is often a sense of being at a family reunion, when attending conferences or through regular work interactions between companies. I am certain that almost every single professional in the CDM world is only two connections away from every other person in this network.

This means that there is a very high likelihood for people interested in your background and reputation, for example when interviewing for a new role, to be able to tap into their trusted network to hear about your past performances and your reputation.

How do you build a good reputation and what does "good reputation" actually mean?

I can tell you from plenty of my own experiences that it does definitely not mean having to execute perfectly every task on every single day, to shy away from tougher discussions, or to always concur with your superiors.

Not just for the purpose of striving for a good reputation in your professional environment, but for many other aspects in life, I did find the following characteristics to play an important role:

- **Accountability:** Own your mistakes! Do not sugarcoat them and do not try to find excuses. Analyze what went wrong, present the facts, and offer solutions on how to fix the issue at hand and how you plan to ensure that the likelihood of a re-occurrence can be minimized.

- From a personal perspective, this was one area I struggled with early on in my career.

- It was Hugh who provided me with feedback that I tended to get very defensive when mistakes happened on my studies. Looking back at the younger Me, I think it was based on a level of insecurity stemming from a real or perceived lack of experience, the fear of disappointing people in your inner circle, and the normal feeling of embarrassment following subpar performances.

- I can also share with you that transitioning from pointing the finger at somebody or something else toward stepping up and accepting accountability is liberating and a key skill required, especially in leadership roles.

- **Trust**: Trustworthiness is another key piece in the Reputation – Puzzle. In essence, trust is following through with actions matching your words. Combining trust with the previous bullet on accountability it means that either you consistently, without exception, actually do what you said you would do, or, if you failed to do what you were supposed to do, you are open about that fact and say that you failed and offer a solution to remediate the situation you caused.

- Failing only once in this approach can cause friction in professional relationships or tarnish your reputation and take a long time to heal. People do remember what you say, and they also know when you did not follow through with your actions.

- **Authenticity:** Trust and authenticity go hand in hand on the life-long journey toward building an extensive network of people, of whom most will speak highly of you, even when you are not in the same room, when you are the topic of discussion. Being your true self, owning your mistakes, accepting your shortcomings and areas of improvement, and not trying to hide them, but accepting them, are huge steps toward opening the trust-door. People in general are pretty good at detecting spuriousness and fakeness, which will make them think what else might not be real about you. There are different ways to cope and address one's weaknesses. In addition to continuing to work toward improving these areas, whatever they might be, I do recommend being open about them. For me personally, I found that in many situations, when my weaknesses are out there for everybody to see, it helped me to not take myself too seriously and apply some humor.

- One short and related anecdote I can share with you is that during an MS-Teams online preparation for a larger CDM virtual town hall meeting my direct reports and I went through the topics we wanted to address. For whatever reason we were not able to turn off the setting in MS-Teams showing the closed captions at the bottom of the screen, while we were speaking. The feature alone can be distracting enough, but especially with a non-native English speaker like me on this call the closed caption rendition of our spoken words turned out to be hilarious. Yes, on the one hand it was embarrassing to see in writing which English words I consistently failed to pronounce properly but on the other hand just accepting the reality that there are words I cannot pronounce and having this bonding experience with my team and having some good laughs was priceless. It makes you human. For the record, it turns out that my absolute nightmare word is "squirrel".

Leadership and Legacy

Picking up where we left off on my career journey, we will now enter the final period and bring us to the present day.

After only 15 months at that Biotech in Maryland, where I was leading a small CDM department as Senior Director, Hugh Donovan took another significant gamble with me by offering me a global VP position in his Global Data Operations department at one of the leading CROs in the world.

Until then I had spent my entire career, about 23 years, at sponsor companies and I truly did not see myself moving over to the service provider side of our industry. However, Hugh had been able to bring together some colleagues from the previous company, where we worked together, and some other phenomenal individuals, to form a very strong leadership team. The prospect of eventually realizing one career goal of mine that had started forming in my head in recent years, to lead a larger global team, and the feeling that I just simply had to trust Hugh and follow his call again, led me to accepting the role of VP of Database & Statistical Programming, overseeing a team of 600 people, and reporting to Hugh directly.

I did feel bad about leaving that Biotech company after such a short time, when I clearly had not been able to finish the job I had started there, in terms of transforming the CDM team into a fully respected and integrated department that can add value beyond the task of providing listings to be reviewed by clinical. Luckily, the Head of Biometrics and my small team were nothing but fully supportive and understanding of the career step I had decided to take.

Starting at that global CRO in a VP Role and for the first time on the service provider side was similar to my move into the new US environment more than a decade earlier. Even though I had had ample experience in dealing with CROs and technology providers in my previous roles, being on the inside now meant having to learn many new things very quickly. The major difference that became apparent after just a few days was the hyperfocus on the financial aspects of the company and the business at hand.

Yes, managing costs, having to justify new headcount, or finding support for new initiatives were common tasks working on the pharma and biotech side as well; however, in the new environment the emphasis on metrics such as "billability", "utilization" for the individuals, or very ambitious revenue targets for the department were new concepts for me.

This final part is about leadership. In my previous roles, leadership primarily meant to provide subject matter expertise, build and organize the CDM teams to be as prepared as possible to execute the studies at hand, and yes, try to inspire and develop people, by creating growth opportunities for them.

In addition to the leadership tasks I was used to, new areas to step in as a global department head emerged quickly.

Let us look at some of these leadership components, which in my opinion are typical when moving from middle management roles to VP+ positions:

- Leading a diverse, large, and global team
- Culture and values
- Dichotomy of Executive Leadership goals and the employee's goals and interests
- Moving from tactical to strategic approaches

Leading a Diverse, Large, and Global Team

When I joined this large CRO in 2014, the database and statistical programming team was about 600 people large with the majority of staff located in India, China, Taiwan, South Africa, Germany, Russia, England, and the US. I inherited a mix of tenured regional directors for the different areas in my department and was looking forward to getting to know them individually together with their respective teams.

Trying to learn from previous mistakes at other companies, I intentionally gave myself about 2 months to spend most of this time just listening through either virtual or in person one-on-one meetings, small group settings, or larger departmental townhall meetings in the different office locations around the globe.

Key takeaways I want to share with you, which I felt were beneficial to start building trust with my global team, are: go back to the previously discussed items of authenticity and start creating a foundation and cultural environment that allows trust to grow. How did I do this?

Firstly, when visiting one of our offices, I made sure that it was not just planned as a 1-day visit, with the main agenda items being a large town hall meeting and a handful of closed-door meetings with other VPs or Directors.

The minimum amount of time I aimed to spend in any given location was 3 full business days and longer when possible.

A typical 3-day agenda looked like this:

- Day 1: Small group meetings with all the managerial staff, a few one-on-ones, and, most importantly, small role-specific group meetings with individual contributors in an informal setting. And, if open timeslots remained, an open-door session, which allowed people to just show up in my temporary office to chat. Lastly, an after work social/fun event.
- Day 2: Time for the town hall meeting, which now I was able to slightly adjust, if needed, by ensuring weaving in topics of interest expressed on Day 1.
- More informal small group meetings and more time for open-door sessions, as well as meeting local leaders from other departments. Another social/fun after work event, if possible, with the entire team.

- Day 3: Completing final small group sessions, ensuring that every person on my team in that office had a chance to interact with me in the town hall meeting, a small group setting (8–10 people), or during the open-door sessions individually. A wrap-up meeting with the local management team to provide feedback on observations I had made during those 3 days and agree on the resulting action items for all of us.

Following this template, which is basically an emulation of what I had seen Hugh do when he came to Frankfurt as Head of Biometrics, seemed to be working well. I do have to emphasize though that choosing this approach was certainly not intended in a manipulative way by playing nice or presenting myself differently than I would do in a different business setting or outside of work.

The truth is that I genuinely was looking forward to hearing what everybody had to say, I was truly enjoying meeting all of these individuals, which ultimately were the main contributors for the success of the company, and I always felt it to be a privilege and honor to interact and learn from my team directly.

It was not a checklist item on my to-do list; I wanted to be there.

Still remembering how I felt earlier in my career with less experience and in an individual contributor role, when an executive was visiting our office. There were those who were welcoming and easier to connect with and other individuals, who seemed to be surrounded by an aura of unapproachability.

Even if you are an individual who is not focused at all on titles, degrees, or levels, new work acquaintances do not know this about you from the get-go and might still find it difficult to open up.

It has to be felt by the employees around you that you are creating a safe space to speak freely and that everybody has a voice and will be treated fairly. Respectful disagreements need to be welcomed, as they will spark healthy debates and create new perspectives and a more vibrant and trusting work environment.

As I am writing these words, I wonder how obvious a thought this is for you, or if you can think of examples in your own career, when you directly by your title and level, being either "higher" or "lower" on the totem pole, felt a disconnect and barrier between you and your counterpart.

This paragraph can be summarized with some key principles:

- Bring your expertise and enthusiasm to the meeting, but leave your title at the door
- An outsider observing one of your group meetings should not be able to identify easily who the department head is
- Be authentic and show vulnerability

I want to share a few more career-defining moments with you during my 4 years at that CRO, which will shed some light on the "Legacy" part of this section.

Based on the constant need for new resources in my department and the push from the finance team and executive leadership to bring costs down, I started to explore Academy Programs. These were initiatives where we would engage with universities located close to our global offices to introduce clinical research to students in their senior year with degrees suitable for roles in our industry.

We did so with SPU (Shenyang Pharmaceutical University) and CMU (China Medical University), for our Shenyang office, Christ University for our office in Bengaluru (India), and with other local universities in Chengdu (China), Taipei (Taiwan), Bloemfontein (South Africa), Sheffield (England), and the US.

I truly enjoyed being able to meet during my periodic office visits with the faculty staff of those universities and engage with students directly to open for them the mostly unknown career paths within Biometrics or other clinical research departments.

It kept on surprising me that these incredibly smart, energized, and ready-to-take-on-the-world graduates were only considering more typical government roles or other more limited career paths.

Being able to open the door for some of these young people and seeing them go through our internal training programs, work on their first studies, and get promoted into more senior roles over time was, and kept on being, truly rewarding. When running those Academy Programs, it did not cross my mind at the time, but in retrospect I do believe that it has been motivated in part by what Oscar Vanderbeke had done for me more than 3 decades ago.

One shift I had noticed in me, after a few years in different VP roles, was that when I had been asked in the past to share my main motivation and satisfaction for being in this industry, my answer was unequivocally to improve people's lives through the discovery of new medicinal products. Even though this aspect always remains the main goal of our industry and is a big part of my motivation, I do feel that finding new talented people, helping them during their early career steps, providing opportunities, and taking risks for them on their growth paths feel even more rewarding.

Not as the main intent, but as a very nice resulting by-product, I do know that these actions are building blocks of creating one's legacy.

This brings us to the second example of a career-defining moment at this first CRO-stop for me – The Executive Leadership Training by Insigniam.

Kudos to the leadership at my company for investing in this extensive Training Program for 21 individuals which were all at VP+ levels and relatively successful in their careers. The entire training program spanned over 8 months, with a total of five sessions of 3 days each, with plenty of assignments throughout the entire time.

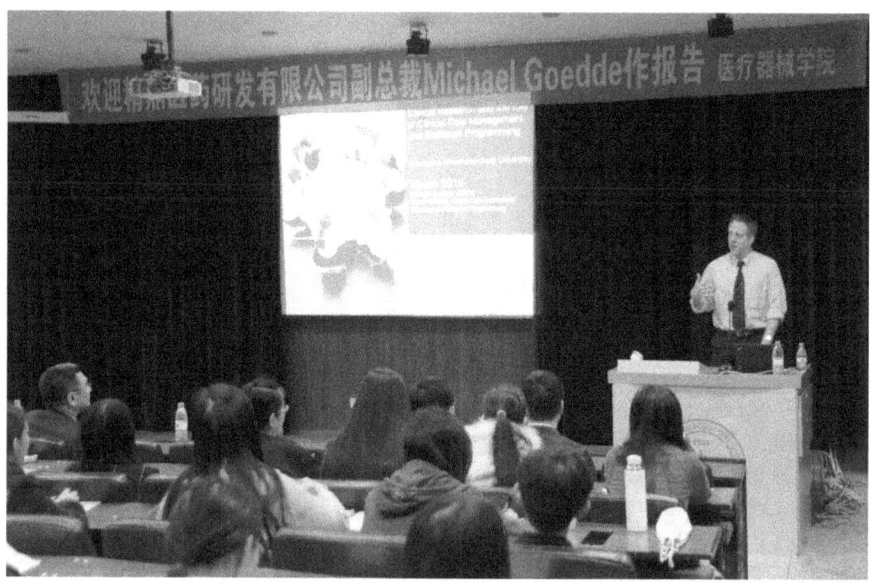

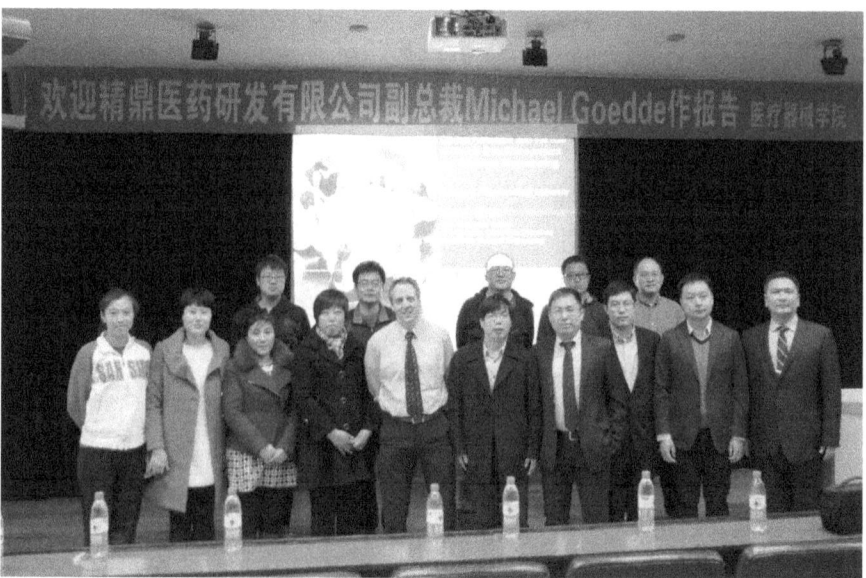

FIGURE 9.3
Scenes of meeting with students and faculty of SPU and CMU in Shenyang (China).

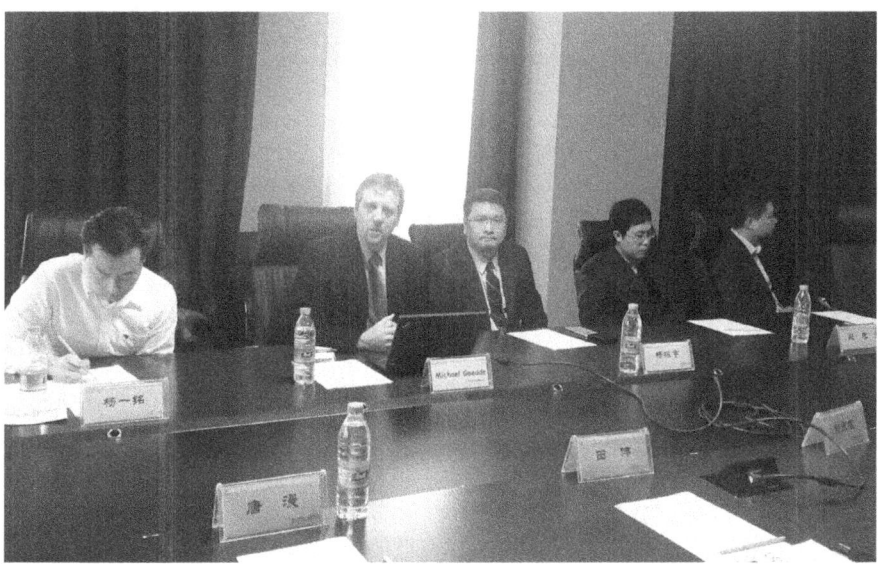

FIGURE 9.3
(Continued)

What made this training unique and so much more valuable compared to anything else I had witnessed until then were the phenomenal trainers we had and the way the entire group of 21 individuals gelled over time.

The exercises became more intense with every session, in terms of getting to the core of our personal struggles, fears, insecurities, and doubts. It was fascinating and inspiring to see industry veteran peers show vulnerability.

The reason I mention this training experience is the fact that it was so eye-opening and grounding to go through some very humbling and vulnerable lessons with the support of your peers. One concrete example that I can share with you was the exercise of writing one's own eulogy. It made you think about how you want people to remember you after you are gone.

Common themes that emerged were to have lived a life that did help and inspire other people, together with the desire to be remembered overall as a good person who in general did not act in a selfish way.

I am certain you can see the parallels between these overall common sentiments and desires, which lie below the surface of our consciousness, and the true objective of being in a managerial or more strategic role.

Yes, in any leadership role, you are obviously accountable for the overall achievement of your departmental goals and the pursuit of continuous improvement of the relevant key performance indicators within your realm.

However, I do see the number one responsibility and duty for anybody in a managerial role, regardless of level, be it an Associate Manager or all the way up to the CEO of the company, to be there for the people in your team.

What does it mean to be there for the people in your team? In my interpretation and actions, it means the following:

- You are open, authentic, and truthful with them. This does not contradict instances when in more senior roles you might be exposed to confidential information, which needs to be treated as such and cannot be shared with your team. People who trust you understand this.
- You care for them on all levels. Meaning professionally and if needed and welcomed also beyond the professional environment with the goal to ensure a healthy work-life balance.
- You put their interests and wellbeing above your own – well above.
- You act as a buffer from the business pressures coming from whatever superior levels and be reassured of the path to take forward.
- You defend your team externally and fix issues internally.
- You listen to any arising concerns, regardless of how small or trivial they might seem to you, and do everything you can to address them.

The insights and hopefully the takeaways from this previous paragraph are leading now to the final example I want to share with you from my first CRO experience.

I want to preface the following by saying that I had more than three very rewarding years at that company and am thankful for the experiences I was allowed to have in my different roles, and the privilege to work with my phenomenal global team.

In my final year a noticeable transformation happened. The focus shifted even more intensely to the financial metrics of the company. The already high scrutiny on metrics such as utilization of employees, which in a nutshell is a measurement of the percentage of time that employees can be billed for their work to customers, was pushed to unreasonable levels. This triggered higher turnover rates as people were not enjoying their work environments as much anymore, which undermined our long-term strategic efforts of the academy programs as an example. Layoffs, mostly motivated just by the desire to increase margins by a few more decimal points, by shifting from seemingly higher cost regions to lower cost regions.

Please do not get me wrong! I fully understand the pressures of a publicly traded company, which must report quarterly numbers influencing stock prices directly. However, I am not willing to put CEO's and Board of Director's main goal of higher stock prices above the care and wellbeing of the people who actually do the work and enable the business to function in the first place.

The concrete event that happened to me, when I felt that I had to move on because the culture had shifted in such a way that made the adherence to the managerial guidance listed earlier, impossible to follow, occurred during a townhall meeting in Hyderabad.

We were in the middle of the annual merit and bonus cycle, and the allocated departmental budgets for distribution were very small. In my opinion, which was also echoed by every other manager in my department, the budget was not proportional to the outstanding performance, business growth, and top-quality work that had been done.

There I was, standing in the big cafeteria room in our Hyderabad office, in front of the more than 250 people my department had at that location, just wrapping up my presentation and opening the typical Q&A part. I was very proud of my team, because they had had another outstanding year. After my frequent visits to the office, they knew that they could speak their mind and ask more direct questions in these town halls – and they did.

First question I got from one of the local managers was: "Michael, sorry for my question, but I do not understand the merit increase budget we just got in relationship with the announcement from our CFO that came out this morning talking about another record year for our company. Can you please explain?"

One second, two seconds, three seconds passed. All the politically correct and corporately approved answers popped into my head, but none of them passed my personal test of authenticity and integrity.

This person, who had the courage to ask a question like this in such a public setting (likely feeling as squeezy as I felt 20 years earlier when I was asking Hugh), did not deserve the cookie cutter answer around the ways CFOs have to speak to the Street to represent our company publicly and what we then do internally.

Why do there have to be two stories for the same thing? If the company did as well as announced, then do take care of the people who made the success happen in the first place and show that we truly are a people-first company.

I thanked the gentleman for his courageous question and he, together with our 250 colleagues in that room, did not get the cookie cutter answer, but my honest opinion and true sentiment about the current state of the culture and values in our work environment.

A few weeks later I resigned from my job at that CRO and joined another global player in the service provider area as VP of Global Data Operations.

At this stage in my career, even though the work environments and roles got more intense, time consuming, and strategic, it did start to feel easier to be considered for VP+ roles in the Biometrics area. I attribute this to everything discussed in this chapter already, especially around the established network I had built, continuous support from mentors and senior leaders who could serve as references, as well as my continuous involvement at industry events.

It was in 2016, when I felt an even stronger desire and need to try to further push and support the CDM profession and decided to run for the BoT (Board of Trustees) position for SCDM. I did get the majority of the votes from the members and became officially part of the SCDM BoT in 2017. After

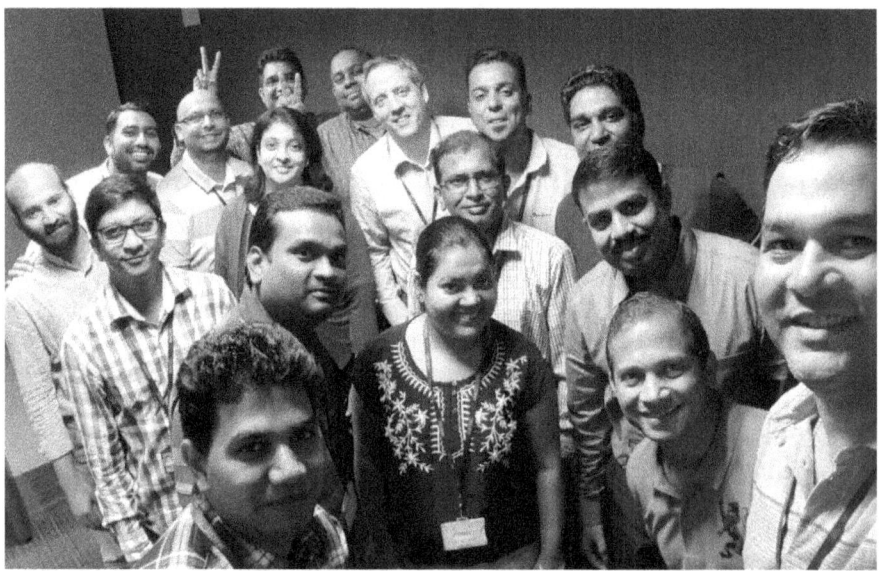

FIGURE 9.4
The outstanding CDM leadership team from Hyderabad I had the privilege to work with Parexel.

my first year on the Board, I was asked to run for the 3-year Officer rotation to become Vice-Chair, Chair, and Past Chair for the Society. I felt honored and slightly overwhelmed but knew deep inside that this was a unique opportunity to truly leave a lasting mark, maybe even a legacy, for a group of professionals that I felt such a strong connection with.

I did get the vote of trust and was elected to become SCDM's Vice Chair, Chair, and Past Chair for the respective years 2019, 2020, and 2021.

It should come as no surprise to you, dear reader, at this stage of your journey with me, that one focal point of my agenda at SCDM was to emphasize the human behind every CDM role, the importance of a people-first culture, and the continuation of seeking new ways to further promote our position in the industry.

Looking again at the topics of leadership and building a legacy, I was able to get support at all three large CROs I worked for, to become the main sponsor of SCDM and through those sponsorships allow everybody in my team and within Biometrics to become a member of SCDM, without incurring any personal costs. To be able to convince my leadership to invest in these activities and sponsorships, opened the door for 100s of people in my respective teams to pursue the certification programs of SCDM, if they wanted to, and to start getting a feeling for the industry forums, the same way I did back in 2004 at my first conference in Toronto.

Now, years later, I see many of my previous colleagues actively involved in these global events and it fills me with incredible joy and pride to see them on stage, in leadership panel discussions, be part of volunteer groups, and become the next generation of industry advocates for CDM.

Wrapping up my career journey, the role of VP of Global Data Operations, was one of my most joyful professional periods. That CRO advocated and lived a people-first culture, despite being publicly traded and having to push for an attractive financial picture.

It started with the CEO and cascaded down to all managerial levels and individual contributors.

Under the leadership of my direct manager, Michael Massaro, who was appointed to oversee Biometrics, the department transformed into the poster child for how to successfully run a global operational team that can grow revenue for the company, while operating within an agreed-upon cost structure, that is not based on the ill-advised and myopic desire to grow margins through cost cutting.

I was also fortunate and felt blessed by feeling the trust from my superiors to develop and build my CDM Leadership Team. Weekly one-on-ones with all my direct reports were events I really looked forward to, even if the agenda was holding more controversial topics. Everybody, without exception, would speak their mind freely, allowing us to analyze situations objectively and allow for the best idea that came up collectively to become reality.

Reflecting on those years, I think I enjoyed that period so much, because, as a team, we helped guide the industry toward moving CDM to CDS. I felt that our department was not just a commodity, but a respected contributor to the overall success of the company. It was understood that having this well-orchestrated global team work cohesively was more valuable than trying to cut costs by going through an Excel-based finance exercise to compare salaries as the main decision maker.

And last, but definitely not least, I personally felt that I was able to open career paths for so many individuals in our team, allowing their talents to flourish. No better feeling than seeing people from your team taking off in their careers.

All great things come to an end eventually, and after another mega merger in the industry between my company and another CRO, I felt that some of that culture eroded and with a similar feeling like the one I had almost 18 years prior, in terms of not seeing a path forward to correct course, I resigned from my job.

That summer I took a break to consider what I wanted to do next in my career. Even though taking multiple months off to reflect on the next steps might not be an option for some of you, I want to encourage you to find periods of time to weigh the pros and cons of your own professional situation. This does not mean to keep changing jobs at the first occurrences of some difficulties, adversity, or a smaller than expected salary increase; however, it does mean evaluating as objectively as possible the following questions:

Am I the right person in my current position to help the company achieve its main goals?

Does the company need my contributions and efforts, while treating and compensating me fairly?

Do I agree with most of the leadership decisions and the overall direction of the company?

Do I like the culture of the company?

If there are items I do not like or do not agree with, do I think I might be able to influence a change for the better?

Depending on how you answer these and similar questions for your own situation, do not be afraid to see what other great opportunities might be out there for you, where your true value and passion are recognized and where you feel that you can make a difference, regardless of how junior or senior your role is.

After a few months of reflection and evaluating different opportunities, which ranged from leading larger global Biometrics teams to possibly starting my own consultancy company, I decided, to the surprise of some, to accept the position of President for Bioforum – The Data Masters, a 200-people Biometrics-focused CRO.

You might ask – why?

One of the main reasons was my instant connection with both Founders, Amir Malka and Eyal Wultz. Two brilliant individuals who could not be more different in their thinking, character, and approach, but together formed a congenial team. After a few meetings with them, I saw the potential value I could bring to Bioforum and by doing so continue my passion of moving CDM, and Biometrics in general, into becoming the focus area of clinical research.

To be clear, both founders also had an agenda to continue to grow the business and increase revenue and margins; however, that goal was not put above all other items. There were many examples shared with me and corroborated by staff how generous Bioforum was in good times and how supportive the company was during tougher times. The positive culture was alive and real.

As I am writing these lines, I am now about 18 months into my Executive Role of President at this company and enjoy the fact of being able to influence the company's strategic outlook, continue to focus on the wellbeing for all of our employees, seek development opportunities for our rising stars, and try to identify the next generation of leaders.

This brings us to the present day and concludes my career journey from the introverted and self-doubting programmer I was more than 3 decades ago to the professional and human I am today. I truly thank you, dear reader, for allowing me to share this personal story with you, in the hope that some of the examples provided can be helpful to you to overcome doubts on your end or make decisions on future career moves more sound.

The journey of CDM is not finished yet. Likely it will never be. We have come a long way as an industry and as a profession, but more work and new challenges are ahead of us. The next generations entering our industry do not have the benefit of the decade-long experiences some of us have, but they undoubtedly deserve to be given the opportunities and freedom to grow to ready us for the clinical research challenges of the future.

I am counting on you to continue the journey for CDM and for the patients who trust us to ensure decisions on new drugs are sound and based on reliable clinical data that You are responsible for to deliver. Enjoy the ride!

Index

Note: Page numbers in *italics* indicate figures and page numbers in **bold** indicate tables on the corresponding pages.

For Product Safety Concerns and Information please contact our EU
representative GPSR@taylorandfrancis.com
Taylor & Francis Verlag GmbH, Kaufingerstraße 24, 80331 München, Germany

www.ingramcontent.com/pod-product-compliance
Lightning Source LLC
Chambersburg PA
CBHW070950200526
45161CB00001BA/64